T0226764

Churchill Livingstone's International Dictionary of Homeopathy

For Churchill Livingstone:

Publishing Manager: Inta Ozols
Project Development Manager: Mairi McCubbin
Project Manager: Jane Shanks
Design Direction: George Ajayi

Churchill Livingstone's International Dictionary of Homeopathy

Prepared in collaboration with the Faculty of Homeopathy and the Homeopathic Trust

Jeremy Swayne BA BM BCh MRCGP FFHom
Dean, Faculty of Homeopathy, London, UK

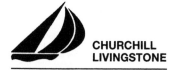
CHURCHILL LIVINGSTONE

EDINBURGH   LONDON   NEW YORK   PHILADELPHIA
ST LOUIS   SYDNEY   TORONTO   2000

CHURCHILL LIVINGSTONE
An imprint of Harcourt Publishers Limited

© Faculty of Homeopathy, UK

All rights reserved. No part of this publication may be reproduced, stored in a retrieval system, or transmitted in any form or by any means, electronic, mechanical, photocopying, recording or otherwise, without either the prior permission of the publishers (Harcourt Publishers Limited, Harcourt Place, 32 Jamestown Road London, NW1 7BY), or a licence permitting restricted copying in the United Kingdom issued by the Copyright Licensing Agency, 90 Tottenham Court Road, London W1P 0LP.

First published 2000

0 443 06009 6

British Library Cataloguing in Publication Data
A catalogue record for this book is available from the British Library

Library of Congress Cataloging in Publication Data
A catalog record for this book is available from the Library of Congress

Note
Medical knowledge is constantly changing. As new information becomes available, changes in treatment, procedures, equipment and the use of drugs become necessary. The author and the publishers have, as far as it is possible, taken care to ensure that the information given in this text is accurate and up-to-date. However, readers are strongly advised to confirm that the information, especially with regard to drug usage, complies with the latest legislation and standards of practice.

Transferred to digital print 2007

Printed and bound by
CPI Antony Rowe, Eastbourne

The Publisher's policy is to use **paper manufactured from sustainable forests**

Contents

Editorial Committee

Chief editorial adviser

Dr Peter Fisher MA FRCP FFHom
Clinical Director, Royal London Homoeopathic
Hospital, London, UK

Committee

Dr Dean Crothers MD
Medical Director, Evergreen Center for Homeopathic
Medicine, Edmonds, Washington, USA

Dr Med. Ing. Friedrich Dellmour
Research Fellow, Ludwig Boltzmann Institut für
Homöopathie (Graz); Coordinator, Subcommittee
Pharmacology, Materia Medica and Pharmacopoeia,
European Committee for Homoeopathy (Brussels),
Feldkirchen, Austria

Professor Flávio Dantas
Head of the Department of Clinical Medicine,
Federal University of Uberlândia, Uberlândia-MG,
Brazil

Professor Edzard Ernst MD PhD FRCP(Edin)
Director, Department of Complementary Medicine,
University of Exeter, UK

Dr Edoardo Felisi
Scientific Director, Centro Italiano di Studi e di
Documentazione in Omeopatia, Milan, Italy

Dr Peter Fisher MA FRCP FFHom
Clinical Director, Royal London Homoeopathic
Hospital, London, UK

viii **Editorial Committee**

Dr Jonathan Marchand MB BCh(Rand) MFHom(UK)
Co-founder Faculty of Homoeopathy of South Africa,
Johannesburg, South Africa

Wenda Brewster O'Reilly PhD EdM
Independent Author and Editor Palo Alto, California, USA

Bernard Poitevin MD PhD
President of the French Association for Research in
Homoeopathy, Editor of L'Homéopathie Européenne,
France

Dr D P Rastogi MA DMS MBSHom DFHom
Consultant Physician, Boeninghausen Academy Clinic,
Surajkund Haryana; Past Director, Central Council for
Research in Homeopathy, India

Dr Jeremy Swayne BM BCh MRCGP FFHom
Dean, Faculty of Homeopathy, London, UK

Special editorial advisers

Dr Steven B Kayne PhD MBA DAgVetPharm FRPharmS FCPP
Pharmacy
Consultant Homoeopathic Pharmacist, Pharmacy Tutor
to the Faculty of Homeopathy, Academic Departments,
Glasgow Homoeopathic Hospital; Visiting Lecturer,
University of Stathclyde, Glasgow, UK

Dr Bernard Leary MR CGP FFHom
Biography and history
Honorary Librarian, Faculty of Homeopathy, London,
UK

Mrs Mary Gooch MIIS
Librarian, British Homoeopathic Library and
Hominform, Academic Departments, Glasgow
Homoeopathic Hospital, Glasgow, UK

Additional Contributor

Dr Harald Gaier
Homeopathic and Naturopathic Practitioner and
Author, UK

Contributors to the European Commission Homoeopathic Medicine Research Group (HMRG) dictionary

European Commission HMRG: steering committee

Dr Peter Fisher
Clinical Director, Royal London Homeopathic Hospital, London, UK

Professor Edzard Ernst
Department of Complementary Medicine, University of Exeter, UK

Dr John English
Faculty of Homeopathy, London, UK

Professor Jochen Mau
Director, Institute for Statistics in Medicine, Heinrich Heine University, Dusseldorf, Germany

Consultants from the European Union and affiliated states

Spain
Dr Xavier Cabré
Member of Academía Médica Homeopática de Barcelona, Spain

Italy
Dr Carlo Cenerelli
Italian vice-president, Liga Medicorum Homoeopathica
Internationalis, Italy

Netherlands
Dr Elly de Lange de Klerk
Homeopathic physician and researcher, Netherlands

Greece
Dr Alexandra Delinick
Research Director of Athenian Center of Homeopathic
Medicine, Greece

Republic of Ireland
Dr Brian Kennedy
Member of the Faculty of Homeopathy,
London, UK

Germany
Dr Walter Köster
Author and authorised teacher of homeopathy,
Germany

Portugal
Dr Alda Pereira da Silva
Graduate in Homeopathy, University of Bordeaux,
France, and Faculty of Homeopathy, UK

UK
Mr Tony Pinkus
Homeopathic Pharmacist, London, UK

France
Dr Philippe Servais
President of Groupe d'Étude d'Homéopathie Uniciste,
Paris; Professor of Institut National d'Homéopathie
Français, France

Norway
Dr Aslak Steinsbekk
Research board of Norske Homeopaters
Landsforbund; Editor Homøopatisk Tidsskrift,
Norway

Belgium
Dr Michel van Wassenhoven
Belgian Vice-President, Liga Medicorum
Homoeopathica Internationalis; Belgian Delegate to
COST B4 EU Program

Germany
Dr Frank Wieland
Co-ordinator of ECH Subcommittee Drug Provings,
Member of Homoeopathic Medicine Research Group,
Co-author of the Guidelines for Research in
Homoeopathy, published by the Commission of the
European Communities, Directorate General XII

Preface

In the 200 years of its history, homeopathy has spread to most regions of the world with the exception of eastern Asia. In the process its philosophy, principles and practice have been affected by different influences and undergone a number of changes. The result is a diversity which sometimes divides its practitioners and teachers and which can render the subject doubly obscure to the rest of the medical world and to the general public. Consequently, this dictionary has been written with three audiences and three purposes in mind. Its purposes, as with any dictionary, are to define, clarify and inform. For students and practitioners of homeopathy, clarification demands a process of growing consensus. This was inherent in the origin of the Dictionary (see Introduction), and will continue to be reflected in this and subsequent editions. The style of the dictionary is therefore unusually discursive, using a comment section to elaborate many of the definitions and to point out areas of uncertainty and differences of opinion. Our intention has been eclectic: we have included concepts that reflect different doctrines and different therapeutic approaches, without presuming to judge their relative merits.

At the time of writing, the mechanism of action of homeopathic medicines remains to be elucidated. Although their effectiveness is accepted by many, especially in parts of the world where homeopathy is well established, such as India and South America, their efficacy has still to be proved satisfactorily to medical science. There is much to be explained and much to remain sceptical about although there has been rapid progress in research, particularly clinical research, in recent years. Nevertheless, these difficulties are more likely to be overcome if there is a better awareness and understanding of the subject within medicine and among the general public. The Dictionary's purpose to define, inform and clarify is therefore directed to these two audiences as well as to students of homeopathy.

I would like to thank the Editorial Boards for all their work on this project and Michael Dean for his substantial contribution to the dictionary, as copy editor.

London, 2000   Jeremy Swayne

Introduction

Origin and development of the Dictionary

The forerunner of this dictionary was an initiative of the Homoeopathic Medicine Research Group (HMRG), an expert group supported by Directorate-General XII (Science, Research and Development) of the European Commission. The composition of the HMRG was balanced, including doctors who practise homeopathy, doctors and medical scientists who have conducted clinical and non-clinical research in homeopathy and an approximately equal number of experts in a range of medical sciences including pharmacology, clinical pharmacology and biostatistics, who were sceptical about homeopathy. The group was drawn from many member states of the European Union. The Dictionary was one element of a programme intended to lay the foundation of the Commission's enquiry into homeopathic medicine.

There have been other dictionaries of homeopathy, but the European Commission project had two particular advantages. The first was its collaborative nature. The work involved representatives of several EU member states, both in the planning and management of the project, and in developing the content of the Dictionary. This collaborative process has been continued, indeed strengthened, in the development of the new work by the appointment of the present international editorial committee to carry on where the European group left off. A few members of the committee are drawn from the European group, and others of that group have made contributions to the new work. The word 'international' is sometimes used in the title of publications to lend undeserved authority. In this case its sense is absolutely literal. There has been extensive collaboration over the composition of definitions and comments and, as the editorial committee makes plain, the contributions have been truly international, and representative of a number of schools and versions of homeopathy.

The second advantage of the original work was the opportunity to develop it in an evolving and dynamic manner. The first version of the Dictionary was of necessity limited both in scope and in depth. The available time and money did not permit the level of research and consultation needed to achieve an authoritative and definitive consensus, and the work emphasised the need for continuing critical debate about the use and meaning of many key concepts. The mechanism for this had yet to be worked out at the time, but it became possible through the commitment of Churchill Livingstone as publishers on the one hand, and the Homeopathic Trust on the other.

This new dictionary is not itself the end of the process, however. Often it does not resolve the differences and uncertainties, but makes them more explicit. It still does not pretend to be complete or definitive. New contributions, criticism and debate have been received up to and beyond the deadline for completion, and material for the next edition is already in hand. This is appropriate if the Dictionary is to be a living stimulus to the growing understanding and authority of this most challenging and exciting medical discipline. Our intention will be well served by feedback and criticism from readers from within and without the homeopathic community. You are invited to contribute, and advice on doing so is displayed on page **xxv**.

Our hope is that this dictionary will achieve wider circulation and greater use, and contribute to consensus among the international homeopathic community on the essential principles and practice of homeopathy. Where differences of opinion and uncertainty exist, we hope that they will act as stimuli for investigating, clarifying and reconciling these issues. As the Dictionary evolves we hope to include or provide access to a bibliography for users to extend their enquiry. The development of an electronic version will further assist the growth of clarity and precision in homeopathy.

We believe this dictionary represents a major advance in defining the conceptual framework of homeopathy. It does not remove all the problems: many involve medical and scientific questions which will be resolved only by further research; many relate to still unresolved philosophical or doctrinal differences, or differences of opinion about clinical method; some arise at the interface between homeopathy and other complementary therapeutic methods and diagnostic techniques with which homeopathy may be combined or confused. Defining concepts is an essential preliminary to identifying and clarifying the problems, which is in turn essential to resolving them.

The scope of the Dictionary

The Dictionary is intended, first, to give the reader an understanding of the language of homeopathy and its most important concepts, particularly those that form the common currency of its contemporary teaching and practice; second, to explain these within their historial context, provided by historical and biographical entries, and historical data within other entries; third, to relate, where necessary and appropriate, concepts from homeopathy to concepts in conventional medicine.

Biography and history
Only individuals who have died have been included. Brief biographies are given of men and women who have had a significant role in shaping the development of homeopathy, or whose lives illustrate its development; the same principles have been applied to the selection of historical events. The inevitable disagreement about where the line has been drawn will be debated during the preparation of future editions.

Organisations and institutions
Very few are included, because of difficulty in deciding criteria for their inclusion. Again, consideration will be

given to including a more comprehensive selection in a future edition.

The language of the Organon
There is a great richness of ideas and terminology in **Hahnemann's** writings which, although they are important for the fuller study of the subject, are not part of the common currency of the language of homeopathy today. This edition of the Dictionary does not attempt to reflect them. The glossary and index of the edition of the **Organon** listed among the sources and references examine these in context in a way that the Dictionary could not have done.

Repertory language
Students of homeopathy encounter difficulty with the archaic language of the repertories (see **repertory**). However, this terminology is of relevance only to users of the repertory in clinical practice, and is not important to an understanding of homeopathic principles and practice. It is not included here, but it is one of the subjects of Yasgur's dictionary, listed in the Sources and Bibliography.

Research terminology
The European dictionary which was the precursor of this book was commissioned to include a large section of research terms. Only those few are retained which are central to the research effort in homeopathy. Other sources are more appropriate for those who wish to explore the terminology of research methodology.

Conventional medical terminology
Despite the conceptual and philosophical differences from mainstream medical thought which are demonstrated here, homeopathy is usually practised within a framework of **conventional** medical thought and practice. Except in developing countries, where conventional drug treatment may be unavailable, doctors and statutorily registered health care professionals who practise homeopathy integrate their homeopathic practice with other interventions – conventional and **complementary** – and treat aspects of

patients' health status and health care needs to which homeopathy, or homeopathy alone, is not appropriate. The extent to which **non-medically qualified homeopathic practitioners** do so depends on the individual practitioner and the degree of regulation or lack of it that exists in the region where they practise. But the conventional diagnosis and treatment is, or should be, at least part of the frame of reference. There is therefore no absolute divide between the language of homeopathy and conventional medicine. The latter, of course, is not within the remit of this dictionary, but some conventional terms are included where they illuminate or lend perspective to concepts from homeopathy.

Other therapeutic and diagnostic methods
A number of therapeutic methods may be associated or confused with homeopathy. For example, it is often mistakenly believed to be a form of **herbal medicine**, and **biochemic medicine**, **Bach flower remedies** and **anthroposophical medicine** have some common features, but differ in important respects. Where there is sufficient common ground, such therapies have been included. Others, which often combine homeopathic medicines with diagnostic techniques which have nothing to do with the homeopathic method, have not been included. Amongst these are dowsing and radionics. One exception is the **vega machine**, because it is often employed to select homeopathic medicines by practitioners who also use homeopathy in the traditional manner.

Spelling conventions
The spelling of 'homoeopathy' with three 'o's, which has been the convention in the UK hitherto, has been changed to omit the second 'o' except in titles where tradition requires that it should be retained. In all other instances the now more widely accepted spelling, 'homeopathy', which has been adopted by the Faculty of Homeopathy, the Homeopathic Trust and the British Homeopathic Journal, has been used.

Similarly, in line with contemporary usage, Greek forms of words such as 'aetiology' are given with 'e' instead of 'ae' as the preferred spelling, cross-referenced to the Greek form.

The structure of the dictionary

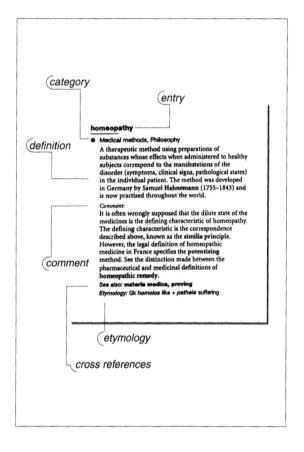

category

entry

definition

homeopathy

● Medical methods, Philosophy

A therapeutic method using preparations of substances whose effects when administered to healthy subjects correspond to the manifestations of the disorder (symptoms, clinical signs, pathological states) in the individual patient. The method was developed in Germany by Samuel Hahnemann (1755–1843) and is now practised throughout the world.

Comment:
It is often wrongly supposed that the dilute state of the medicines is the defining characteristic of homeopathy. The defining characteristic is the correspondence described above, known as the *similia* principle. However, the legal definition of homeopathic medicine in France specifies the potentising method. See the distinction made between the pharmaceutical and medicinal definitions of **homeopathic remedy**.

comment

See also: materia medica, proving
Etymology: Gk *homoios* like + *patheia* suffering

etymology

cross references

Categories and the category index

The first line following each main entry assigns the term to one or more categories, which are listed with all the terms in each category in the category index at the end of the book. The categories are not intended to be a classification; they provide a descriptive overview, offering the reader different views of the subject matter. The purpose of this is to provide a conceptual framework for readers who are unfamiliar with homeopathy to explore the subject, and to allow readers to browse selectively among terms related to one aspect of it.

Many terms appear a number of times in different categories. Thus, for example, the appearance of **chronobiology** in the *Physiology* and *Symptomatology* categories draws attention to the timing and cyclical nature of biological events, not only as a physiological phenomenon, but as a significant aspect of the study of patients' symptoms.

Definition and comment

Many entries include a section of comment, following the definition. This has a number of purposes. One is to give the concept a wider *perspective*. Examples include **Avogadro's number**, where its significance for homeopathy is emphasised, and **clinician**, where the various uses of the term are described. Other perspectives which may be provided include the historical context and the development of homeopathic thought or practice.

The comment section also highlights *inconsistencies* or *differences* of opinion or usage, in keeping with the dictionary's aims of clarification and consensus. An example is the entry for **classical homeopathy**.

A third use is to point out the *relationships* between different concepts. Examples are **clinical homeopathy**, where the relationship to classical homeopathy is explained, **allopathy**, where the comparison with homeopathy and other treatment methods is made, and

alternative medicine, where the distinction between alternative, complementary and integrated medicine is highlighted.

Cross-references

Extensive cross-referencing between entries is provided. Many terms in an entry need to be explained themselves if the entry is to be fully understood. Those terms that have their own entries in the dictionary are given in **bold** type. In addition, many entries will be understood better if studied in the context of other related or contrasting concepts. These contextual references to other terms are given as *See* in the text, and in the *See also* note following the main entry.

Synonyms and alternative terms

Synonyms are listed immediately after a main entry. Synonymous terms, alternative terms which are not precisely synonymous, and closely related terms which are not themselves defined but are encompassed by another main entry, have their own alphabetical place in the Dictionary with the annotation *See* identifying the main entry.

Etymology

The etymology of terms has been given selectively, where it seems necessary or of particular interest. Abbreviations used for etymological entries are as follows:

AF	= Anglo-French		Heb	= Hebrew
F	= French		L	= Latin
f.	= from		LL	= Late Latin
Ger	= German		ME	= Middle English
Gk	= Greek		OE	= Old English
Gmc	= Germanic		OF	= Old French

The future of the dictionary

The intention to develop the scope and authority of the dictionary over successive editions has already been made plain. This development will be significantly influenced by feedback from readers. Whatever your interest in the subject, and whatever your degree of enthusiasm or scepticism, **you are invited to contribute to this process**.

How should the dictionary be expanded and developed? What criticisms do you have of its content or style? What are its errors and omissions? How can it help more effectively to identify the need for consensus, and to achieve it? How can it help to identify the research objectives necessary both to prove and to improve homeopathy? How can it help to establish the role of homeopathy in the spectrum of medical care? **We would like to hear from you**.

Comment and criticism may be sent by post to:
>   **Dictionary of Homeopathy,**
>   **The Faculty of Homeopathy,**
>   **15 Clerkenwell Close,**
>   **London EC1R 0AA**

or by e-mail to:
>   **indichom@btinternet.com**

or via the Faculty website:
>   **www.trusthomeopathy.org**

a

accessory symptom

● Symptomatology

1 A minor symptom; a symptom that is not **pathognomonic**.
2 A symptom that is incidental (secondary, supplementary, subordinate) to the **presenting problem**. Accessory symptoms are those which may occur in conjunction with particular presenting symptoms, forming a cluster of symptoms.
   See also: **concomitant symptom, incidental symptom**

activity

● Pharmacology and drug action

1 The property of an agent (in this context a medicine) to stimulate change in a biological system.
2 The change stimulated by an agent in a system.
   See also: **drug action, reactivity, receptivity**

acute case

● Case taking and analysis, Disease processes

1 The record of a patient with an acute **illness**.
2 The patient who presents with an acute **illness**.
   Etymology: L *acutus* p.p. of *acuere* sharpen, or *acus*

acute disease

● Disease processes

A pathological process which may vary in intensity,

but which has a rapid onset and limited duration. Ending in resolution, either spontaneous or in response to treatment, or in death.

Comment:
See **disease** and **illness** for comment on the distinction between the two.

See also: **acute illness**

Etymology: L *acutus* p.p. of *acuere* sharpen, or *acus*

acute illness

● Disease processes

An **illness** with a rapid onset, an intense course and a limited duration.

Comment:
1 In homeopathy an acute illness is often seen as a manifestation of an underlying **chronic** trait. An acute epidemic disease may arise as an isolated phenomenon.
2 See **disease** and **illness** for comment on the distinction between the two.

See also: **acute disease**

Etymology: L *acutus* p.p. of *acuere* sharpen, or *acus*

acute remedy

● Materia medica, Therapeutics

Homeopathic medicine indicated in an **acute case**, particularly in a specific **acute illness**, or during the acute phase of a **chronic disease**. These medicines generally have shorter duration of action, or exhaust their action relatively quickly, and so may require frequent **repetition of the dose** to achieve the desired result.

See also: **remedy**

Etymology: L *acutus* p.p. of *acuere* sharpen, or *acus*

adjuvant

● Pharmacology and drug action, Pharmacy, Therapeutics

An ingredient that facilitates or modifies the action of the principal ingredient of a medicine. For example, the vehicle used in formulating an injection may have an effect on its dispersal within tissues or body fluids.

Comment:
It is postulated that the alcohol–water vehicle may act as an adjuvant in facilitating the action of **potentised** homeopathic remedies. One possibility is that the structure of solvent molecules may be electrochemically changed by **succussion**, enabling it to acquire an ability to 'memorise' an imprint of the original remedy (see **information medicine hypothesis, memory of water**).

See also: **excipient**

Etymology: L *ad- + juvare,* pres. p. *-juvans,* to help, give aid to

adjuvant therapy

● Therapeutics

The use of one treatment to assist and complement another. Chemotherapy and radiotherapy are sometimes described as **adjuvant** in the treatment of cancer.

See also: **compatible, synergism, complementary**

administration of the medicine

● Therapeutics

Act of administering a medicine to the patient, as distinct from prescribing or dispensing the medicine.

See also: **route of administration**

adverse drug reaction (ADR)

● Disease processes, Therapeutics

A reaction which is harmful and which occurs at doses of the drug normally used in humans for prophylaxis, diagnosis or therapy or for the modification of physiological function. For example, bleeding from the stomach due to aspirin, and hemorrhage due to anticoagulants.

ADRs are usually classified as type 1 or dose-dependent and type 2 or idiosyncratic. Type 1 reactions are relatively common, varying in severity between individuals, but proportional to the dose. Type 2 reactions are much rarer, occurring in a small proportion of people who take a drug, typically producing stereotyped syndromes which may occur in response to a very small dose.

Comment:
Although it is believed that no harm can result from the **specific effects** of homeopathic medicines, the following effects can be distinguished:

1 **Pathogenetic** symptoms if the medicine is taken for too long or repeated too frequently, when symptoms characteristic of the medicine may occur, resolving when the medicine is withdrawn.
2 **Therapeutic aggravation** of the existing symptoms, although indicating a favourable response and usually well tolerated, may be intense or prolonged.
3 The transient increase in symptoms that may be brought about by a **similar** medicine that is not the **simillimum** and which does not lead on to an improvement in the patient's condition.
4 **Hypersensitivity** or toxic reactions can occur if very **low potencies** or **mother tinctures** are taken, especially in large doses or if repeated frequently.
5 Type 2 reactions may be compared to **proving** reactions in sensitive **volunteers**.

See also: **complication, risk, sensitive type**

aetiology, aetiological

See: **etiology, etiological**

affect

See: **emotion**

affinity

● Materia medica, Therapeutics
1 Similarity suggesting relationship.

2 Liking for; attraction between.
3 Relationship between medicines; sometimes implying **synergism** or complementarity.
4 Relationship between medicines and their main region of action (e.g. **organ affinity, tissue affinity**).

See also: **disease affinity**

Etymology: L *affinitas* bordering on

after action

See: **counteraction**

aggravating factor

● Disease processes, Symptomatology

A factor which causes an existing state to become worse. May be external circumstances or an event internal to the patient (such as another **symptom**). External factors include **conventional** and **homeopathic medicines**.

Comment:
Factors which aggravate or **ameliorate** symptoms are important **indications** in homeopathic prescribing and are known as **modalities**.

See also: **aggravation, therapeutic aggravation, precipitating factor**

aggravation

● Disease processes, Symptomatology
1 Increase in severity, worsening, of the illness.
2 Increase in severity of symptoms in response to external events, circumstances or activities, or to an event internal to the patient such as change in body function or another symptom (e.g. headache worse during stool), or to the administration of a medicine or other therapeutic intervention.

Comment:
The term aggravation may be synonymous with

exacerbation in both conventional and homeopathic usage. In conventional use, however, exacerbation implies a change for the worse in the course of the disease, by contrast with the transient increase in symptoms in response to the homeopathic prescription, which usually carries a good prognosis (**therapeutic aggravation**).

See also: **aggravating factor, amelioration, exacerbation, modality**

Etymology: L *aggravare* to make heavy (*gravis*)

ailments from . . .

● Disease processes, Materia medica, Symptomatology

1 Describes the role of etiological factors in the onset or **evolution** of illness, often the role of emotions and the emotional impact of life events but also such things as disordered body functions or environmental factors.

2 Many homeopathic medicines are associated with specific **etiology** of this kind. This association is often described by a **rubric** or epithet beginning 'ailments from . . .' Such a clear attribution of **causality** is important in the **evaluation of symptoms**.

See also: **etiological factor, etiological prescribing, aggravating factor, modality, never well since, precipitating factor**

Allen, Henry C

● Biography

Canadian homeopathic physician (1836–1909). Served as professor at a number of homeopathic medical schools. With Swan he described the first proving of **lueticum.** His works included *Keynotes of the Leading Remedies,* and *The Materia Medica of the Nosodes.*

See also: **keynotes, materia medica, nosode**

Allen, Timothy Field

● Biography

American homeopathic physician and teacher (1837–1902). Compiler of the *Encyclopedia of Pure*

Materia Medica. This described symptoms derived from **provings** and omitted any based solely upon clinical experience.

allergen

● Disease processes, Physiology

Foreign material capable of provoking **allergy**.

See also: **antigen, allergode**

Etymology: Gk *allos* other + *ergon* work + *genes* born

allergode

● Pharmacy, Therapeutics

Homeopathic remedy derived from source material known to cause an **allergic** reaction (e.g. grass pollens or house dust).

See also: **isopathy**

Etymology: Gk *allos* other + *ergon* work + *eides* like

allergy

● Disease processes

1 **Hypersensitivity** reaction.
2 An acquired overreaction of the immune system to repeated exposure to a foreign material, not of itself harmful, by contact, inhalation or ingestion, causing local or systemic disorder.

See also: **idiosyncrasy, sensitivity, tolerance**

Etymology: Gk *allos* other + *ergon* work

allopathic

● Medical methods, Pharmacology and drug action, Philosophy, Therapeutics

Pertaining to **allopathy**.

allopathic medicine

● Medical methods, Pharmacology and drug action, Philosophy, Therapeutics

Literally methods of medical treatment based on

allopathy. However, the term was used by
Hahnemann, and is still commonly but
incorrectly used to describe all other forms of
mainstream **conventional medicine**, not only
allopathy.

allopathy

● Medical methods, Pharmacology and drug action,
Philosophy, Therapeutics

Treatment whose action has no direct relationship to
(is other than) the effects of the **illness**, the
symptoms. The effects of the drug or treatment
method bear no relationship to the symptoms or
other effects of the illness. ('Neither similar nor
opposite, but quite heterogeneous to the symptoms
of the disease.' – *Organon* §22 (1)) For example,
the use of electroconvulsive therapy to treat
depression.

Comment:
The term was invented by Hahnemann to describe one
of the four therapeutic methods that he distinguished
in successive editions of the *Organon* and to
differentiate his new system of therapeutics from the
mainstream medical practice of his day. The other
three methods were: (i) the **homeopathic** method,
'similia similibus curentur', in which the pathogenic
effects of the source material are *similar* to the effects
of the illness: (e.g. Belladonna to treat the kind of
intense fever with rapid onset similar to its toxic
effects – see **scarlet fever**); (ii) the **antipathic,
enantiopathic** or **palliative** method, ' **contraria
contrariis curentur**', in which the action of the
conventional drug is the direct *opposite* of the effects
of the illness (e.g. codeine phosphate, whose primary
effect is to cause constipation, to treat diarrhea); and
(iii) in the posthumous sixth edition, the **isopathic**
method in which the pathogenic agent responsible for
the illness is used to treat it (e.g. pollens in hay fever).
Hahnemann did not finally approve of isopathy
although he experimented with it.

Synonym: **heteropathic medicine**
See also: **allopathic medicine**
Etymology: Gk *allos* other + *patheia* suffering

alternating remedy

⬤ Therapeutics

Intercurrent use of a homeopathic medicine to support the use of another.

Comment:
Despite **Hahnemann's** general insistence on the doctrine of the single remedy, the use of medicines in alternation was introduced by him to increase the action of repeated doses of the same medicine, if a single dose is not powerful enough to cure the patient in **chronic diseases**. During the 19th century there was much argument about whether he had authorised the alternation of medicines. In Britain in the second half of the century alternation was commonplace, at least for **acute** conditions.
See also: **intercurrent remedy, following remedy**

alternating symptoms

⬤ Case taking and analysis, Disease processes, Symptomatology

Symptoms which appear in alternation. Both are features of the patient's condition, but only one is present at any one time. When one appears the other remits, and vice versa. For example, asthmatic respiration alternating with urticaria is an indication for the homeopathic medicine *Caladium* according to **Kent's repertory**.
See also: **metastasis, syndrome shift**
Etymology: L *alternare* do things by turns (*alter* one or other of two)

alternation

See: **alternating remedy**

alternative medicine

● Medical methods

Beliefs about health and illness, and approaches to diagnosis, prevention or treatment which have not been developed by generally accepted scientific methods.

Comment:
This term has been widely superseded by the term **complementary medicine** or **integrated medicine** to avoid the implication that 'alternative' and conventional methods are necessarily mutually exclusive. The two terms are often combined as 'Complementary and Alternative Medicine' (CAM).
Etymology: L *alter* one or other of two

amelioration

● Healing processes, Symptomatology

1 Reduction in the extent or severity of the illness or of particular symptoms.
2 Reduction in severity of symptoms in response to external events, circumstances or activities, or to an event internal to the patient such as change in body function (e.g. abdominal distension relieved by passing wind) or another symptom (e.g. headache relieved by nosebleed), or to the administration of a medicine or some other therapeutic intervention.

Comment:
Aggravating factors and factors which ameliorate symptoms are important indicators in homeopathic prescribing and are known as **modalities**.
See also: **aggravation, therapeutic aggravation**
Etymology: F *ameliorer* f. OF *ameillorer* (*meilleur* f. L *meliorem* better)

American Institute of Homeopathy

● History

First national homeopathic medical organisation in

the United States. Founded in 1844, it had two
essential purposes: to reform and augment the
materia medica, and to restrain physicians from
pretending to be competent to practise homeopathy
who have not studied it in a careful and skilful
manner. Constantin **Hering** was elected the first
president. It was the first national medical association
in America with regulatory purpose. In 1847 the
American Medical Association was formed in part as a
response to it.

See also: **Flexner report, Simmons**

analogy

● Philosophy, Therapeutics

Similarity, correspondence or resemblance (to, with or
between).

Comment:
Occasionally used as an alternative to **similarity**.
Etymology: GK *analogia* proportion

anamnesis

● Case taking and analysis
1 Calling to mind; recollection.
2 Patients' account of their **illness** and health **history** in
its historical and biographical context.
3 Process of enquiry to elicit the story of the illness from
the patient.
Etymology: Gk *anamnesis* remembrance
See also: **case taking**

antagonist

● Pharmacology and drug action, Physiology

Agent that counteracts (opposes, impedes or
neutralises) the action or effect of another within the
body. Examples range from the action of one muscle
in counterbalancing another, to a drug blocking a
receptor site.

See also: **antidote, inimical**

Etymology: Gk *anti* against + *agon* contest

anthroposophical medicine

● History, Medical methods, Philosophy

Medicine of the knowledge of man. Philosophy and system of medicine based upon the insights and teachings of Rudolph **Steiner** with the assistance of Dr Ita Wegman, relating to the spiritual nature of human existence. It is a therapeutic method which includes the use of some medicines derived from the homeopathic **materia medica**, not prescribed according to the **similia principle**, but using 'spiritual science', the **doctrine of signatures** and metaphysics. Preparation of the medicines does involve **dilution** with rhythmic agitation, but not the same process of **succussion** used in homeopathic pharmacy to achieve **potentisation**.

Etymology: Gk *anthropos* man + *sophos* wise, *sophisma* argument

antidote

● Pharmacology and drug action, Therapeutics

1 Commonly, any substance or procedure used to counteract the effect of a poison; literally a thing 'given against' another.

2 Used in homeopathy to describe the action of one medicine inhibiting or counteracting the effect of another, or of any other substance counteracting the effect of a medicine.

Comment:

1 The effect of an antidote may be to slow down, arrest or reverse the action which it opposes.

2 Three general types of antidotes to the action of homeopathic medicines can be distinguished: (i) physical antidotes (e.g. hot or cold applications, compresses, massage), (ii) chemical antidotes (e.g. coffee, alcohol, camphor, spiritus nitri dulcis), also

known as **diadotes,** and (iii) dynamic antidotes (e.g. homeopathic medicines chosen according to actual symptoms), also known as **homeodotes.**

3 The evidence that the chemical antidotes described above do inhibit homeopathic medicines is inconclusive.

See also: **antagonist, inimical**

Etymology: Gk *anti* against + *doton* given

antigen

● Disease processes

Substance capable of stimulating a specific immune response in a host organism to which it is foreign.

See also: **allergen**

Etymology: Gk *anti* against + *genes* born

antihomotoxic therapy

● Medical methods, Therapeutics

Detoxification with homeopathic medicines in high potency.

See also: **homotoxicology, toxins**

Etymology: Gk *anti* against + *homos* the same + *toxa* arrows *(toxikon pharmakon* poison for arrows)

antiluetic

See: **antisyphilitic**

antipathic

● Pharmacology and drug action, Philosophy, Therapeutics

Antagonistic to, of contrary nature to the disease; pertaining to methods of treatment whose primary effect is directly opposite to the effects of the **disease.** For example, the treatment of diarrhea with codeine phosphate, whose primary effect is to cause constipation.

Comment:
One of the four therapeutic methods described by
Hahnemann, the others being the homeopathic, the
allopathic and the isopathic. See **allopathy** for a
discussion of these. The antipathic method is
sometimes confused with the allopathic.
Synonyms: **enantiopathic, palliative**
See also: **contraria contrariis curentur**
Etymology: Gk *anti* against + *pathos* suffering

antipraxy

● Pharmacology and drug action, Philosophy

A theory of the action of homeopathic medicines
propounded by Dr William Sharp (1805–1896) and
other homeopathic physicians of the day, which states
that all medicines in larger and smaller doses produce
opposite effects, the smaller dose actually opposing the
disease process which the larger dose will cause. This is,
arguably, the **antipathic** principle, not the **homeopathic**.
See also: **Arndt-Schultz law, dose-dependent reverse
effect, hormesis, organopathy**
Etymology: Gk *anti* against + *praxis* doing, action

antipsoric

● Materia medica, Therapeutics

1 Homeopathic medicine used to treat a **syndrome** or
clinical picture attributable to the **psoric miasm**.
2 Homeopathic medicine whose **materia medica**
approximates to that described for **psora**.
Synonym: **homeopsoric**
See also: **miasm, diathesis**

antisycotic

● Materia medica, Therapeutics

1 Homeopathic medicine used to counteract a syndrome
or **clinical picture** attributable to the **sycotic miasm**.
2 Homeopathic medicine whose materia medica
approximates to that described for **sycosis**.

Synonym: **homeosycotic**
See also: **miasm, diathesis**

antisyphilitic

● Materia medica, Therapeutics

1 Homeopathic medicine used to counteract a syndrome or **clinical picture** attributable to the **syphilitic miasm**, a concept introduced by Hahnemann which is related to, yet different from the modern concept of syphilitic infection and pathology.

2 Homeopathic medicine whose **materia medica** approximates to that described for 'syphilis'.

Synonym: **antiluetic, homeosyphilitic**
See also: **miasm, diathesis**

antitaxic drug action

● Pharmacology and drug action

The action of a drug in dilution which is opposite to its action in standard dose.

See also: **Arndt-Schulz law, biphasic activity, dose-dependent reverse effect, hormesis, simillimum**

Etymology: GK anti against + taxis order

apothecary

● History

Archaic title for modern day pharmacist or druggist. In **Hahnemann**'s Germany apothecaries had the sole legal right to prepare and dispense medicines. This brought them into conflict with Hahnemann who not only prepared and dispensed his remedies but made no charge for them.

approved indication

● Therapeutics

Well-tried and reliable indications for prescribing a particular medicine. Not 'approved' in the sense of 'authorised'.

apsoric

- Materia medica

  Medicines that do not pertain to the **psoric miasm**, as opposed to those used to treat it (**antipsoric**).

Arndt-Schulz law

- Physiology

  States the relationship between the strength of a stimulus and its effect upon physiological activity, namely that (i) weak stimuli encourage living systems, (ii) moderate stimuli interfere with living systems and (iii) strong stimuli inhibit or destroy living systems. The law was formulated by Dr H R Arndt and Professor H Schulz of the University of Greifswald, Germany in the 1880s.

  See also: **antitaxic drug action, biphasic activity, hormesis, dose-dependent reverse effect**

artificial disease

  See: **experimental pathogenesis**

  Etymology: L *ars, art-* put together + *facere* make, do

ascending potencies, ascending scale

- Pharmacy, Therapeutics

  A term used to describe a range of increasingly high potencies, sometimes prescribed as separate but successive doses in a course of treatment.

'as if' symptom

- Case taking and analysis, Materia medica, Symptomatology

  Symptoms described by the patient in terms of some other familiar or imagined subjective experience, e.g. 'it feels as if. . .' or 'I feel as if. . .'. A type of **strange, rare and peculiar symptom** of special interest for **individualisation** of the prescription.

  Synonym: **sensation as if**

  See also: **subjective**

associated manifestations, associated symptoms

See: **concomitants**

attenuation

● Pharmacology and drug action
1 Dilution; reduction in intensity.
2 A reduction in the virulence of a pathogenic organism.

Comment:
Although not strictly accurate, it has been used in place of the terms **dynamisation** or **potency** (as in 'the 6th attenuation'). The US homeopathic pharmacopeia (8th edn vol. 1, 1979) refers to dilutions as liquid attenuations but includes **succussion** in the description of the process.

See also: **dilution, immunisation, potentisation**

aude sapere

● Philosophy
Latin phrase meaning 'dare to know', 'dare to be wise'.

Comment:
1 Inscription on the title page of the ***Organon***.
2 The phrase was probably used first by the Roman lyric poet, Horace. It was later used as a motto summarising the principles of the Enlightenment by the 18th-century German philosopher, Immanuel Kant, who interpreted it as meaning: 'Have courage to use your *own* understanding.'

audit

● Research
1 Detailed and systematic review of data to assess and evaluate a process.
2 Comparison of performance against a previously agreed standard of good practice to identify opportunities for improvement.
Etymology: L *auditus* hearing, *audire* to hear

autocracy

● Philosophy
1   Supreme authority bestowed in one individual.
2   Controlling influence.
3   Term used by **Hahnemann** to clarify the meaning of
    'vital force' (**life force**).

Etymology: Gk *autocrateia* (*autos* self + *kratos* power)

autohaemic therapy

See: **autohemic therapy**

autohemic therapy

● Medical methods, Therapeutics

The administration of **nosodes** prepared from a blood
sample usually obtained from the patient being
treated. Occasionally a pooled sample obtained from
several patients may be used as the source material.

Comment:
1   Further autohemic methods have been developed
    by mixing the patient's blood with homeopathic
    potencies before reinjection, and by various special
    methods such as the incubation of blood with
    ozone or oxygen.
2   Not a common feature of mainstream homeopathic
    practice, but sometimes used for the treatment of
    allergies as an **isopathic** approach; usually an
    adjuvant therapy combined with homeopathy
    (often **combination remedies**), or other
    complementary therapies.

Synonym: **autosanguine therapy**
See also: **autoisopathy, isopathy, autonosode,
homotoxicology**
Etymology: Gk *auto* self + *haima* blood

autointoxication

● Disease processes

Illness caused by the accumulation of **toxins** produced
within the body.

See: **homotoxicosis, drainage therapy**

Etymology: Gk *auto* self + *toxa* arrows (*toxikon pharmakon* poison for arrows)

autoisopathy

● Medical methods, Therapeutics

Treatment using preparations of the patient's own body substances (tissues, excretions, secretions). These are technically **autonosodes,** being the product of the disease process (e.g. a discharge), or affected by it (e.g. the patient's urine). An **isopathic** approach; usually an **adjuvant therapy** with other homeopathic medicines, including **combination remedies,** or other **complementary therapies.**

Synonym: **autopathy**

See also: **autohemic therapy, individualised isopathy, isopathy, nosode**

Etymology: Gk *auto* self + *patheia* suffering

autonosode

● Materia medica, Therapeutics

Nosode prepared from pathological material produced by the patient's own disease process. For example, blood, secretions, urine, warts; or milk from a cow or sheep suffering from mastitis.

See also: **autoisopathy, nosode**

Etymology: Gk *auto* self + *nosos* disease + *eides* like

autopathy

See: **autoisopathy**

autoregulation

● Healing process, Physiology

1 Self-regulation.
2 The natural abilities of the organism for regulation, adaptation, regeneration and defence.
3 Mechanisms by which the organism is capable of self-healing.

Comment:
The phenomenon of autoregulation seems to be the common basis for the different methods of **autoregulatory therapy** or **naturopathy**.
See also: **homeostasis**
Etymology: Gk *auto* self + L *regula* rule

autoregulatory therapy

● Medical methods, Therapeutics

Treatment that depends upon stimulating the organism's natural capacity for **autoregulation**.

Comment:
All forms of **natural medicine**, including acupuncture and homeopathy, and many treatments employed in mainstream medicine claim to promote health in this way. The term 'autoregulatory therapy' may be preferred to **natural medicine** and natural therapy in many instances because it describes more explicitly the 'natural' aspect of the treatment, in contrast to the direct manipulation or control of body function or disease processes with **allopathic** medicines.

autosanguine therapy

See: **autohemic therapy**

auxiliaries

See: **auxiliary medicines**

auxiliary medicines

● History, Therapeutics

Medicines, not strictly homeopathic, used in the 19th century in addition to homeopathic **remedies** and regarded as a betrayal of **Hahnemann** by purists.
Synonym: **auxiliaries**
See also: **half homeopaths**
Etymology: L *auxilium* help

auxiliary substance

● Pharmacy

Substances incorporated into the dosage form to stabilise or improve its properties. For example, the excipients starch, calcium behenate and magnesium stearate are permitted for manufacturing tablets in some pharmaceutical processes.

See also: **vehicle**

Etymology: L *auxilium* help

aversion

● Symptomatology

1 Turning away from.
2 Object of strong dislike.

Comment:
May indicate a disturbance of the patient's equilibrium. Relates to foods, environmental factors, circumstances, situations and activities, and people; any factor which affects the physical or emotional comfort of the individual. Such features may be important in homeopathic prescribing. Not to be confused with **aggravating factors**.

See also: **desire, general symptom, modality**

Etymology: L *ab* away + *vertere* to turn

Avogadro, Count Amedeo

● Biography

Italian professor of mathematical physics (1776–1856) who advanced the physical theory that bears his name, known as **Avogadro's law**.

Avogadro's constant

See: **Avogadro's number**

Avogadro's law

● Biophysics

The theory advanced by **Avogadro** that equal volumes

of all gases under identical conditions of temperature
and pressure contain the same number of molecules.
From this hypothesis other physicists were able to
calculate **Avogadro's number.**

Avogadro's number

● Biophysics

The number of molecules, or any elementary particles
theoretically present in one mole of a substance, which
is estimated to be 6.0225×10^{23}. This number is
calculated from **Avogadro's law** which assumes that
equal volumes of all gases under identical conditions
of temperature and pressure contain the same number
of molecules. A mole, one gram-molecular weight, is
the amount of a substance that contains as many
elementary particles as the number of atoms in 0.012
kilogram of carbon 12.

Comment:

1 Avogadro's number is of interest to homeopathy
   because it specifies the potency at which a remedy
   no longer contains any of the original material
   substance. This may vary from 7c (botanical or
   zoological materials) to 11c or 12c (concentrated
   pure chemical substances, including metals) in the
   centesimal potency scale.
2 In fact it is not possible to detect the physical
   presence of any particle beyond a dilution of
   10^{-18}–10^{-20} with analytical methods currently
   available.

See also: **concentration, Loschmidt's number,
ultramolecular dilution**

b

Bach, Edward

● Biography

Physician (1886–1936) best known for his therapeutic system of flower remedies (see **Bach flower remedies**), and also by homeopaths for his work on the **bowel nosodes**. Studied medicine at Birmingham University and University College Hospital, London, qualifying in 1912. He became assistant bacteriologist at the latter hospital, where he began working on bacterial **vaccines** and published work in orthodox journals. In 1920 he obtained the post of bacteriologist at the Royal London Homoeopathic Hospital. Here his bacterial vaccines against chronic disease, based on contemporary theories of intestinal toxemia, were modified according to homeopathic principles and named the **bowel nosodes**. This work was subsequently continued by John Paterson, a Glasgow homeopathic physician. In the late 1920s Bach gradually conceived a mystical philosophy of disease as due to spiritual error, which emphasised psychological rather than physical symptoms as indications for treatment. He experimented increasingly with plant remedies, developing his intuition to sense their healing properties.

Bach flower remedies

● Medical methods, Pharmacology and drug action, Pharmacy, Therapeutics

A set of 38 medicines developed by **Bach** in the 1930s. They are prescribed on the basis of the patient's emotional characteristics; particularly their emotional response to their illness. The flowers, and their association with particular personalities and psychological states were chosen through research and intuition by Dr Bach. The medicines are prepared by two methods: (i) the sun method for delicate flowers that bloom during the late spring and in the height of summer, which involves partial infusion of the flowers in full bloom in water; (ii) the boiling method for more robust materials, such as the flowering twigs and stalks from trees and bushes and plants that bloom early in the year before there is much sunshine. The supposedly energised solutions obtained by these methods are mixed with an equal volume of brandy as a preservative and further diluted (without **succussion**) to obtain the **stock**. There is no similarity to the principles of homeopathy except the apparent mode of action by the stimulus of some subtle energy. Despite this, both methods are contained in the British Homeopathic Pharmacopeia.

Comment:
Other brands of flower remedies prepared by similar methods but not entitled to use the Bach name have been developed in the UK and several other countries, notably Australia, California and South Africa.

back-action

See: **counteraction**

ball mill trituration

● Pharmacy

Method of **trituration** of solid source materials with lactose as a vehicle unless otherwise prescribed. For decimal potencies, 1 part of the source material and 9 parts of the vehicle are placed in a porcelain pot which contains the appropriate amount of porcelain balls (not precisely specified). The mixing time required to achieve homogeneity is determined by a trial run.

basic product

See: **source material**

beet-sugar

See: **sucrose**

Bernard, Henri

● Biography

Leading French homeopath (1895–1980). He developed **constitutional** theories of homeopathy, building on the work of **Nebel**.

bioavailability

● Biophysics and biochemistry, Pharmacology and drug action
1 The measure of the physiological availability of a drug or other substance in the body.
2 The rate at which and the extent to which a drug or metabolite is absorbed into the bloodstream after administration. Determined by the amount of active drug measured in the blood, or by the magnitude of the pharmacological response.

Comment:
In homeopathy the concept may be applied to the release of the active medicinal property of a substance. For example, an insoluble solid such as gold must be subject to **trituration** in order to achieve the bioavailability of its active properties.

biochemic medicine

● Biophysics and biochemistry, Materia medica, Medical methods, Pharmacology and drug action

Therapeutic method directed at remedying deficiencies or imbalance of inorganic salts assumed to be essential to the health of the organism using

dynamised preparations of these salts in **low potency** (originally 6x, but nowadays also 12x) on the basis of the common symptomatology of the condition being treated rather than **individualisation** of characteristics. The method predates modern concepts of biochemistry.

The German physician Wilhelm **Schüssler** (1821–1898) identified 12 functional medicines to be used in this manner. Later 12 supplementary remedies were added. Schüssler remedies are commonly named **tissue salts**.

Comment:
1 Schüssler was greatly influenced by Virchow's theory of cellular pathology, which asserted that all disease processes originated in abnormalities in the cells.
2 The compounds from which the tissue salts are derived are all also the source of well-known homeopathic medicines, and are used as such in a wide range of **potencies**.

Synonyms: **biochemic tissue salts, cell salts, Schüssler remedies, Schüssler salts, tissue salts**

biochemic tissue salts

See: **biochemic medicine**

biodynamics

● Biophysics and biochemistry

The science of the energy or forces active in living matter and living systems.

See also: **autocracy, bioenergetics, dynamis, life force**

Etymology: Gk *bios* life + *dynamis* power, force

bioenergetics

● Biophysics and biochemistry
1 The study of the transfer of energy (bioenergy) involved in the chemical reactions within living tissues and organisms.

2 The study of the transfer and exchange of such energy between living organisms and between living organisms and their environment.

See also: **autocracy, biodynamics, dynamis, life force**

Etymology: Gk *bios* life + *en* in + *ergon* to work

bioenergy

See: **bioenergetics**

bioinformation

● Biophysics and biochemistry

A hypothetical form of information, other than genetic information, possibly **biophysical** or **bioenergetic**, stored and used in biological systems, and capable of influencing their behaviour.

Comment:
It is suggested that homeopathic medicines may possess properties which cannot yet be measured or analysed, but which transmit information of this kind to the organism to which they are administered. A comparison is made to the type of information stored on a magnetic medium, which similarly cannot be identified until it is 'read' by an appropriate receptor.

See also: **information medicine hypothesis**

biological clock

See: **chronobiology**

biomedical model

● Medical methods, Philosophy

Conceptual framework of mainstream western medicine. A reductionist concept based on biological mechanisms.

See also: **conventional medicine, homeopathy, model**

biopathography

● Case taking and analysis, Disease process

A biographical view of the patient's health history. The

evolution of the patient's present state of health throughout his or her life. The story of the illness.

Comment:
Biopathography sets the present illness in the context of the patient's life events and previous experience of illness. In homeopathy, it applies particularly to the history of the development of the symptoms and the changes effected by the illness which are of potential value in understanding the patient and for the prescription.

See also: **anamnesis, pathogenesis**

Etymology: Gk *bios* life + *pathos* suffering + *graphia* writing

biophysics

● Biophysics and biochemistry

1 The knowledge and methodology of physics and physical chemistry applied to biological phenomena.
2 The study of the physical properties and processes (e.g. electrical, electromagnetic) occurring in living organisms.

biphasic activity

● Biophysics and biochemistry, Pharmacology and drug action

1 Two phases of activity working in opposite directions.
2 The principle that differences in magnitude of a stimulus on either side of a critical threshold may produce opposite effects (stimulation and inhibition) in a biological system. This phenomenon is exemplified in the **Arndt-Schulz law** and in the concept of **hormesis**.

See also: **antitaxic drug action, change in phase, dose-dependent reverse effect**

Etymology: L *bi-* having two + Gk *phasis* appearance

Blackie, Margery Grace

● Biography

Physician (1898–1981), Royal London Homoeopathic Hospital. Great-niece of James Compton **Burnett**. A prescriber mainly of **high potencies** and a disciple of James Tyler **Kent**. She was a lecturer of repute, Dean of the Faculty of Homoeopathy 1964–1979, and Physician to the British Royal Household, 1969–1979. A late interest in research led to her founding the Blackie Foundation Trust. Her only book, *The Patient not the Cure*, was historical and autobiographical, but some of her lectures were transcribed by Elliot and Johnson, after her death, as a book, *Classical Homoeopathy*.

blinding

● Research

The masking of trial treatments in a clinical trial to enhance observational comparability with respect to concomitant therapy and care and assessment of outcome. The usual forms are: (i) single-blind, in which only one party, usually the trial patients but sometimes the trial investigators, is unaware of which is the test treatment and which the **control** treatment; (ii) double-blind, in which both the trial patients and the trial investigator are unaware of which is the test treatment and which the control treatment; (iii) observer-blind, where only the person who assesses and records patient outcome is unaware of which trial treatment the patient was actually allocated to, the test treatment or the control treatment.

Boenninghausen, Clemens Maria Franz von

● Biography

One of the most important and eminent of early practitioners of homeopathic medicine. A Dutch lawyer (1785–1864), later given permission to practise medicine by King Friedrich Wilhelm IV, he was converted to homeopathy when cured of tuberculosis with *Pulsatilla* in 1828. From 1830 he was in regular correspondence with **Hahnemann** and **Stapf**. He was the first to recognise the need for a **repertory** to assist in homeopathic prescribing. The series of repertories written by him between 1833 and 1864 were compiled by **Boger** as *Boenninghausen's Characteristics and Repertory*. His work placed particular emphasis on **concomitant symptoms** and the **relationship of remedies**.

Boericke, William

● Biography

Leading homeopathic physician in the USA (1849–1929). Born in Austria, he began his medical studies in Vienna but qualified in Philadelphia and settled in San Francisco. He became Professor of Homeopathic Materia Medica at the University of California. With Richard **Haehl** he conducted negotiations over many years to obtain the manuscript of the 6th edition of the *Organon*. These finally succeeded in 1920 and it was published in 1921. He also translated **Hahnemann**'s revisions to the 5th edition into English.

Boericke and Tafel

● History

First US homeopathic pharmacy, founded in 1853 by F E Boericke and Rudolph Tafel in Philadelphia, Pennsylvania. They also established the Hahnemann Publishing House.

Boger, Cyrus

● Biography

American physician (1861–1935), who compiled and translated **Boenninghausen**'s *Characteristics and Repertory*. He also published his *Synoptic Key to the Materia Medica* in which he emphasised important similarities of apparently dissociated symptom groups.

Boiron, Henri

● Biography, History

French pharmacist (1906–1994) who, with his twin brother Jean (1906–1996) established Laboratoires Boiron in Lyon. They were responsible for achieving the inclusion of homeopathic medicines in the 8th edition of the French pharmacopeia in 1965.

Boiron, Jean

See: **Boiron, Henri**

Borland, Douglas

● Biography

Physician (1885–1960), London Homoeopathic Hospital. One of the first British students of James Tyler **Kent**, he was an exponent of **high potencies**. His *Children's Types*, a monograph arranging children by **constitutional** groups, has become a classic of homeopathic literature.

bowel nosodes

● Materia medica, Therapeutics

Group of 12 homeopathic medicines identified by Edward **Bach** and further developed by John and Elizabeth **Paterson**. Prepared from organisms obtained by stool culture from patients showing particular patterns of disorder who had responded to particular homeopathic medicines. Prescribed on the indications derived from the **clinical picture** of those patients. Used as medicines in their own right on the basis of their own clinical picture or to reinforce the action of their related group of medicines.

Boyd, William Ernest

● Biography

Physician in Glasgow (1891–1955), also a radiologist and a diplomate Member of the British Institute of Radio Engineers, and member of many learned societies. His experimental work convinced him that homeopathic medicines in **potency** possess electrophysical properties which are detectable and distinguishable. He designed and made an instrument called an emanometer for this purpose. As a result of his research he classified homeopathic medicines by these properties and postulated 12 groups, each of whose members had a relationship one with another. His work was investigated by an independent committee, led by Sir Thomas Horder, which reported favourably to the Royal Society of Medicine in 1926.

See also: **relationship of remedies**

brevilinear constitution

See: **carbonic constitution**

British Homoeopathic Society

● History

Organisation of British homeopathic physicians founded by Frederic **Quin** in London in 1844. Became the **Faculty of Homoeopathy** in 1943.

Burgi's principle

See: **synergism**

Burnett, James Compton

● Biography

British homeopathic physician (1840–1901). He developed the concept of **vaccinosis**. He claimed to have prepared *Bacillinum*, a **nosode** prepared from tuberculous lung tissue, and used it for the treatment of tuberculosis 15 years before Koch introduced tuberculin.

C

C potency

Abbreviation for: **centesimal potency**

C3 trituration

● Pharmacy

1 The first three steps in the process of **potentisation** by **trituration** on the **centesimal** scale. May also be used as the first stage in the preparation of **millesimal potencies**. Insoluble substances are triturated with lactose to 3c before suspension in liquid medium for further dilution.

2 Trituration procedure applied by **Hahnemann** to all types of **source material**, including fresh plants, **expressed plant juices**, mercury, petroleum and other liquids, to manufacture the starting **potency** for the preparation of **LM potencies**.

Comment:
Differences in chemical composition of the starting material may occur between medicines prepared from **mother tincture** and triturated medicines, especially if active compounds of source material are insoluble and do not appear in the mother tincture. In the trituration the whole source material becomes the basis of the medicine.

Synonyms: 3c, 3cH

See also: **fresh plant trituration**

cane sugar

● Pharmacy

Sucrose prepared from sugarcane. A constituent of some homeopathic **dosage forms**.

carbonic constitution

● Constitution, morphology and terrain

Nebel's association of certain characteristics of the homeopathic medicine *Calcarea carbonica* and associated medicines with relatively short, stocky, often obese people, with limited extensibility (hypolaxity) of the joints.

Synonym: **brevilinear constitution**

See also: **constitution, constitutional medicine, fluoric constitution, morphology, phosphoric constitution, sulphuric constitution, typology**

case

● Case taking and analysis

1 An occurrence of an illness or disease in a patient.
2 The complete record of the history and management of the patient's problem.

See also: **anamnesis, biopathography, case taking, history**

case analysis

● Case taking and analysis

1 The process of determining the best course of management of a **case**.
2 In homeopathy, the process of finding the best prescription or prescribing strategy by studying the **evolution** of the case; by identifying and evaluating the **characteristics** of the **clinical picture**; and by correlating these with **materia medica** information, which may or may not involve the use of a **repertory**.

See also: **anamnesis, case taking, evaluation of symptoms, history**

case study

● Case taking and analysis

The study of a **case** and the **case analysis**.

case taking

● Case taking and analysis

The process of eliciting and recording the **case** or **history**. Sometimes described as the **anamnesis**.

causal factor

● Disease processes

1 Factor relating to cause.
2 Factor (condition, agent, act etc.) actively contributing to the state that ensues. May be hereditary or any event following conception.

See also: **etiology, causality, causation, causative**

causality

● Disease processes

1 The attribution of cause. The relation of cause and effect.
2 In homeopathic **case analysis**, the attribution of particular significance to certain events or experiences associated with the **onset** and **evolution** of the illness. A clear attribution of causality is important in the **evaluation of symptoms**.

See also: **etiology, causal factor, causation, causative**

causation

● Disease processes

Causing; producing an effect.

See aslo: **etiology, causal factor, causality, causative**

causative

● Disease processes

Active as a cause; the agent which produces an effect. As in 'causative organism', the organism causing an infection.

See also: **etiology, causal factor, causality, causation**

cell salts

See: **biochemic medicine**

centesimal potency

● Pharmacy

1   A **dilution** in the proportion of 1 part in 100.

2   The sequential addition of 1 part of the **stock** or of the previous **potency** to 99 parts of diluent. The number of these **serial dilutions**, performed with **succussion**, defines the centesimal potency. The potencies are designated by a number with the letter 'c' following it. Thus 6c represents a 1:99 dilution carried out serially 6 times, with succession at each stage. A single c or the designation 'cH' indicates that it is a **Hahnemannian potency**. Where no letter is given after the potency number, the 'c' is implied. Examples of centesimal potencies are given below:

Dilution	Concentration	Contesimal potency
1/100	10^{-2}	1c or 1cH
1/10 000	10^{-4}	2c or 2cH
1/1000 000	10^{-6}	3c or 3cH
1/10^{12}	10^{-12}	6c or 6cH
1/10^{30}	10^{-30}	15c or 15cH
1/10^{60}	10^{-60}	30c or 30cH
1/10^{400}	10^{-400}	200c or 200cH

Comment:

1   In fact, the method by which the first potency (a '1c') is made, the precise proportions of the first dilution, varies according to the instructions of the **pharmacopeia** which is followed.

2   The higher potencies (dilutions) are often prepared by the **Korsakov** method. For this reason, the 'm' potencies are written 'mK' in some countries. It is less precise than the Hahnemannian method because molecules of the original **source material**

may persist due to adhesion to the walls of the single glass container in which the potencies are prepared.

See also: **centesimal trituration, LM potency, millesimal potency, potency scale, single glass method**

Etymology: L *centum* a hundred

centesimal trituration

● Pharmacy

Trituration in the proportion of 1 part in 100. Homeopathic **potencies** of insoluble **source materials** are prepared by grinding them with lactose as a centesimal trituration. Insoluble substances are triturated to 3c (**centesimal potency**) before being suspended in a liquid medium for further sequential dilution.

See also: **C3 trituration, centesimal potency, dilution, suspension**

Etymology: L *centum* a hundred

centre of the case

● Case taking and analysis, Philosophy, Symptomatology

The heart of the matter; the fundamental source of the illness in the individual patient; that which is to be treated; the core problem to which the treatment must be directed, and which the choice of homeopathic medicine must reflect. Usually psychological.

See also: **case analysis, case taking essence, theme, Wesen**

cH potency

● Pharmacy

Hahnemannian centesimal; **centesimal potency** prepared by the **Hahnemannian potency** method.

See also: **cK potency**

change in phase

● Biophsics and biochemistry, Pharmacology and drug action

1   The critical threshold between two phases of activity.
    The point of transition from one phase to the other.
    The critical threshold at which the transition between
    phases occurs is known as the change over.
2   The point of transition between the **low dose effect**
    and the **high dose effect**.

    See also: **antitaxic drug action, Arndt-Schultz law,
    biphasic activity, dose-dependent reverse effect,
    hormesis**

characteristic

● Symptomatology
1   Distinctive; typical.
2   Distinctive feature; feature typical of the thing or
    person.

    Comment:
    It is those symptoms or features of the patient which
    are most characteristic of the individual and of the
    individual expression of the **disease** or **illness** in that
    patient that are most important in selecting the
    correct homeopathic prescription.

    See also: **evaluation of symptoms, individualisation,
    pathognomonic**

    Etymology: Gk *kharacter* stamp, impress

chemotherapy

● Medical methods, Pharmacology and drug action,
    Therapeutics
    Treatment which uses and depends upon the direct
    chemical action of the drug in the body. Particularly
    used in cancer treatments but applies to most
    conventional drugs currently in use.

    Comment:
    Whereas homeopathic medicines may be said to have
    a pharmacological action, they cannot be said to be a
    form of chemotherapy when diluted beyond
    Avogadro's number.

    See also: **pharmacology**

chief complaint

See: **complaint**

china, china bark

See: **cinchona**

cholera

● Disease processes, History

An acute water-borne epidemic infectious disease caused
by the bacterium *Vibrio cholerae.* (Originally a
non-specific term for various gastrointestinal
disturbances.) The disease was unknown outside Asia
until 1817 when it spread out of India reaching
Astrakhan in Russia in 1823 and Europe by 1829. By
1831 it had affected Hungary, Poland, Germany and
Britain and was soon transported to America. Further
epidemics occurred in Europe in 1848–9, 1853–5
and 1866. After a period of quiescence, when it
was largely confined to S. Asia, it reemerged in the 1960s,
and is now endemic in Africa and Latin America also.

The use of homeopathy in the treatment of cholera was
an important early demonstration of the **effectiveness**
of homeopathy. In **Hahnemann's** time cholera was
often fatal with allopathic treatment. The mortality rate
was the same under **allopathy** as in untreated cases. In
1831 Hahnemann published his opinions upon the
causation and treatment of the disease. He suggested
that it was transmitted by a microorganism and that in
the early stages it could be cured by *Camphor.* Later
stages required *Cuprum* or *Veratrum album.* Homeopaths
who followed this advice achieved much more favourable
results than their allopathic colleagues. In 1854 the
Governors of the **London Homoeopathic Hospital**
decided that during an epidemic only cholera cases
would be treated, and 90 patients received treatment
with 17 deaths, a mortality rate of 19%. This compared
with an overall rate of 46% in the same epidemic. The
official return recording this success was suppressed by

the Medical Council which had been asked by
the Board of Health to evaluate the effectiveness of
different treatments in cholera. A parliamentary
question eventually led to the publication of
the homeopathic results.

chronic

● Disease processes

Lasting a long time; lingering.

Etymology: Gk *khronos* time

chronic disease

● Disease processes

A **disease** whose onset is usually gradual, which
progresses slowly and whose course is of long
duration with no likelihood of recovery; may consist
of recurrent acute episodes or **exacerbations**; often
involves more than one body system.

Comment:
The concept of chronic disease has particular
significance in homeopathy, since first introduced by
Hahnemann in *Chronic Diseases* (1828–30, 2nd edn
1835–7). He attributed the phenomenon to a deep-
seated trait in the patient which he termed **miasm** and
which requires a particular therapeutic approach.
According to him, chronic diseases are those which (each
in its own way) dynamically disturb the living organism
often gradually and, at first, almost imperceptibly.
Unaided, the **life force** is unable to extinguish the disease
and allows it to develop, progressively undermining the
life force until finally the organism is destroyed.
Hahnemann differentiates between protracted,
longstanding diseases (which include, but are not limited
to, the chronic diseases) and truly chronic diseases. He
attributes true chronic diseases either to chronic miasms
or to the effects of **allopathic** treatments. (Hahnemann
1996 p 294) after WBO

Etymology: Gk *khronos* time

chronobiology

● Physiology, Symptomatology

The study of the timing of biological events, especially repetitive or cyclical phenomena in individual organisms, such as **circadian rhythm** (24-hour **periodicity**). These time patterns are important **characteristics** of the **clinical picture** and of the **materia medica** of homeopathic medicines.

Etymology: Gk *khronos* time + *bios* life + *logos* word, reason, study

cinchona, cinchona bark experiment

● History

While **Hahnemann** was translating **Cullen**'s *Treatise on Materia Medica* in 1790 he disagreed with the explanation of the action of Peruvian bark (cinchona, the source of quinine) in intermittent or marsh fever (malaria). He took repeated doses of the medicine himself and found that he developed many symptoms of the fever. This led him to recognise the remarkable similarity between the symptoms cured by the drug and the symptoms caused by it in his healthy organism during the experiment, and thereafter to develop his **similia principle**: *similia similibus curentur* (let like be cured by like). In 1796 he published his observations together with a comprehensive literature review, which demonstrated that many physicians had previously described similar effects of drugs in diseased and healthy subjects. Consequently, homeopathy is generally considered to have originated at this date.

Synonym: **china, china bark, quinine**

circadian rhythm

● Physiology

Rhythmic variation in biological function with a cycle of about 24 hours.

See also: **chronobiology**

cK potency

● Pharmacy

Centesimal potency prepared by the **Korsakov** method.
See also: **cH potency, potency scales**

Clarke, John Henry

● Biography

British physician (1840–1901), consultant at the
London Homoeopathic Hospital, he was for many
years editor of the *Homoeopathic World*. He quarrelled
with Richard **Hughes** whom he accused of pandering
to the conventional profession and using only **low
potencies**. He welcomed the introduction to Britain of
Kent's prescribing method, with its emphasis on
constitutional features. He was a major contributor to
the homeopathic literature, his best-known works being
*The Prescriber, The Dictionary of Practical Materia
Medica*, and its accompanying *Clinical Repertory*. He
was also active in extreme right-wing political circles.

classical homeopathy

● Philosophy, Therapeutics
1 Doctrine or school of homeopathic philosophy and
  therapeutics claiming to be based on strict
  Hahnemannian principles.
2 Therapeutic method using a single medicine in a
  single prescription. Sometimes associated with the
  unicist school of homeopathy.

Comment:
There is continuing examination of and debate about
Hahnemann's principles and methods; how strict and
consistent these were and whether they provide
justification for identifying a clearly definable 'classical'
tradition. Some interpretations of classical homeopathy
certainly refer to concepts originated by **Kent** rather
than Hahnemann. There is no single agreed meaning of
this term in international homeopathy. It is adopted
with some degree of flexibility by different schools and

practitioners; by some **pluralist** prescribers as well as unicists for example. It is sometimes used to differentiate prescribers who adopt homeopathy as the only medicinal therapy allowed to their patients.

See also: **clinical homeopathy, mongrels, repetition of dose, single dose**

clathrate

● Biophysics and biochemistry

A molecular lattice. The structure of a chemical compound in which molecules of one component are enclosed within the lattice-like structure of another. This phenomenon provides one hypothesis of the mechanism of transmission of the active properties of the homeopathic medicine during **potentisation**.

See also: **cluster, solvation structures**

Etymology: Gk *klethra* lattice-bars

cleaning, cleansing

● Pharmacy

The procedure for removing all traces of previous materials, including previous solutions, or pre-existing homeopathic activity from the utensils used at each stage in the preparation of a homeopathic medicine.

Comment:
It is believed that this cannot be achieved by rinsing alone, but only by superheated steam or heat sterilisation.

clinical

● Case taking and analysis, Medical method, Therapeutics

Pertaining to the observation and treatment of patients; in its literal sense, applies to such activity at the bedside.

Etymology: Gk *klinikos* (*kline* bed), *klinike techne* clinical art

clinical experiment

See: **randomised controlled trial**

clinical homeopathy

● Philosophy, Therapeutics

School of homeopathic philosophy based mainly on **guiding symptoms** and on the predominant correspondence to somatic symptoms, **organ affinities**, **tissue affinities**, **disease affinity**, **etiological prescribing** and **specifics** (so called 'approved indications', German: 'bewährte indikationen').

Comment:
This therapeutic method should be distinguished from **classical homeopathy**, but in practice there are many overlaps between both philosophies. The method is used sometimes by classical homeopaths if the patient's symptoms show a very clear indication according to the approaches mentioned above; but the method is also used by physicians without a detailed knowledge of homeopathy and by patients without medical education (e.g. *Arnica* in bruising, or *Drosera* in cough). It is a specialised use of the term, which might otherwise simply distinguish it from 'academic' homeopathy.

See also: **clinical**

clinical picture

● Case taking and analysis, Symptomatology

Description of all the features of the **illness** – **particular**, **general** and **mental** – in the individual patient.

See also: **clinical, disease picture, drug picture, picture, symptom picture**

clinical trial

● Research

A comparative clinical study; a clinical experiment.

See also: **clinical, randomised controlled trial**

clinician

● Practitioners

Practitioner professionally involved in medical care.

Comment:
As well as doctors, UK dentists, nurses, other therapists and vets, and German Heilpraktiker, are also regarded as clinicians; this is not the case in other EC states where the concept only includes medical doctors.

Etymology: Gk klinikos (kline bed), klinike techne clinical art

cluster

● Biophysics and biochemistry

Aggregation of molecular complexes in liquids. In water and other liquids the single molecules may aggregate to larger molecular complexes like $(H_2O)_2$, $(H_2O)_3, \ldots (H_2O)_n$, which can be distinguished by their physical properties.

Comment:
Although these clusters are unstable and exist only for very short periods, some hypotheses suggest that they explain the storage of **information** in water, ethanol or other vehicles.

See also: **clathrate, information medicine hypothesis, memory of water**

colloid

● Biophysics and biochemistry, Pharmacology and drug action

Submicroscopic particles, aggregations of atoms or molecules, in a finely divided state (the dispersed phase), dispersed in a gaseous, liquid, or solid medium (the dispersion medium); not susceptible to sedimentation, diffusion, or filtration, and thus differing from **suspensions**.

Comment:
Insoluble source materials may pass through a colloid

phase in the preparation of homeopathic medicines
after trituration with lactose.

Etymology: Gk *kolla* glue

combination remedies

● Pharmacy, Therapeutics

Combinations of two or more homeopathic medicines
which are prepared from more than one stock and
incorporated into one dosage form. These medicines
are generally **complementary remedies**. They may be
used in an attempt to treat more than one condition at
the same time.

Synonym: complex remedies

See also: **complex homeopathy, group remedies,
single remedy**

compatible

● Materia medica, Therapeutics

1 Consistent with.
2 Able to coexist with, to be used in combination with.
3 Homeopathic medicines which may be used in
   association with one another with no harmful
   interaction or other disadvantage, but without
   synergistic effect.

See also: **alternating remedy, antidote,
complementary remedy, concordances, inimical**

complaint

● Case taking and analysis, Symptomatology

The problem – symptom, discomfort, distress or
disorder – that the patient presents to the practitioner.
The **presenting problem**. Sometimes used to mean the
illness or **disease**.

Synonym: **chief complaint**

complementary

● Medical methods, Therapeutics.

Making complete.

Etymology: L *complere* to fill up + *-ment* the means of

complementary medicine

● Medical methods

A broad term encompassing 'Those forms of treatment which are not widely used by the **orthodox** health-care professions, and the skills of which are not taught as part of the undergraduate curriculum of orthodox medical and paramedical health-care courses.' (British Medical Association 1993) It has been defined elsewhere as 'diagnosis, treatment and/or prevention which complements mainstream medicine by contributing to a common whole, by satisfying a demand not met by orthodoxy or by diversifying the conceptual frameworks of medicine' (Ernst E et al. 1995).

See also: **alternative medicine, complementary, integrated medicine**

complementary remedy

● Therapeutics

1 Homeopathic medicine whose action may be **compatible** with or **synergistic** to another if used as part of the same regime.

2 Homeopathic medicine representing the **acute** manifestation of a deeper and more **chronic** state, or conversely representing the deeper state underlying an acute manifestation.

See also: **compatible, complementary, concordances, following remedy, relationship of remedies**

complementary therapy

● Medical methods

1 Any one form of treatment used to complement, and integrated with others.

2 A form of unorthodox treatment used to complement mainstream medical care, falling within the broad area of **complementary medicine**. It involves cooperation between treatment methods, as distinct from **alternative medicine** which implies mutually exclusive methods of treatment.

See also: **adjuvant therapy, complementary, conventional medicine, integrated medicine, orthodox**

complete symptom

● Case taking and analysis, Symptomatology

A **symptom** described in all its aspects – localisation and extension, quality or appearance, quantity or severity, timing, **modalities**, setting in which it occurs, associated manifestations (**concomitants**), **etiology** and meaning – is called 'complete symptom' of particular value for choosing the homeopathic medicine.

See also: **evaluation of symptoms, symptom selection, weighting of symptoms**

Etymology: L *complere* to fill up

complex homeopathy

● Pharmacy, Therapeutics

Method of homeopathic treatment using **combination remedies**.

See also: **pluralist homeopathy, unicist homeopathy**

complex remedies

See: **combination remedies**

compliance

● Research, Therapeutics

1 In physiology, the measure of elasticity or distensibility of a structure.

2 In clinical practice, the patient's acceptance of and adherence to the prescribed regime. The degree to which the patient cooperates with and carries out instructions given as to treatment, self-care, lifestyle. (In this context it has recently been suggested that the term 'compliance' suggests

coercion, and that the term 'concordance' is more
appropriate.)
3 In clinical research, the subject's and the
experimenter's acceptance of and adherence to the
protocol.

complication

● Disease processes, Therapeutics

1 A complicating circumstance.
2 A secondary disease; a new disorder occurring
during the course of a disease that is not an
essential part of it. It may be a consequence of
the disease (e.g. bronchopneumonia as a
complication of coma), or have some other cause.
3 An adverse event directly attributable to a specific
medical intervention.

Comment:
Adverse events resulting directly from the use of
homeopathic medicines are claimed to be rare in
clinical practice. Preliminary data suggest that they
are, but more detailed and specific investigation is
required.
See also: **adverse drug reaction, aggravation,
hypersensitivity, idiosyncrasy, risk, therapeutic
aggravation**
Etymology: L *cum* with + *plicare* to fold (+ *-ation* the
result of)

concentration

● Pharmacy, Pharmacology and drug action

The quantity of a specific substance per unit volume or
weight of a more complex substance of which it is a part.

Comment:
The concept of concentration may be applied to the
actual or theoretically calculated amount of source
material in a homeopathic potency.
See also: **Avogadro's number, toxicity, ultrahigh
dilution, ultramolecular dilution**

concomitant symptoms

> *See:* **concomitants** or **associated manifestations**

concomitants

● Case taking and analysis, Symptomatology

1   Things that go together.
2   Symptoms associated with other **symptoms**, appearing at the same time or during the course of the same **disease process**. For example, diarrhea during menstruation, anger when in pain.
    Synonyms: **associated manifestations, associated symptoms**
    See also: **accessory symptom**
    Etymology: L *comes* companion

concordances

● Materia Medica, Therapeutics

1   Things that are in agreement, harmonious.
2   Relationships between homeopathic medicines, first described by **Boenninghausen**. Groups of medicines showing affinity to one another, which may be used in succession in a course of treatment, and which may promote progressive improvement in a case when used in sequence. Similar tables of relationships were created by Gibson **Miller**, **Clarke** and some French authors (Zissu, Demarque).
    See also: **alternating remedy, antidote, compatible, complementary remedy, following remedy, relationships of remedies, synergism**
    Etymology: L *concordare* to be of one mind

constitution

● Constitution, morphology and terrain, Philosophy

1   The constituent parts, composition or make up of a person or thing.
2   The whole pattern of psychological and physical

characteristics, hereditary or acquired, that identify an individual; the imprint of heredity, life events, lifestyle and environment upon the individual.

3 The **health** or strength of the body; the **vitality** and resilience of the individual in the face of any threat to health or wellbeing.

Comment:

1 In homeopathy the constitution describes the psychological and physical characteristics, and reactions to stimuli and circumstances that are found in everyday life in the healthy individual, as compared with these characteristics when affected by **illness** or **disease**, when they contribute to the **totality of symptoms**.

2 The question whether the individual constitution is fixed for life or can change, or be changed by treatment, is a matter for debate.

3 The distinction between constitution and **terrain** is a fine one. It is generally agreed that the terrain can change, or be changed by treatment.

4 The concept of constitution in homeopathy is related to the observation that some **provers** (volunteers in **homeopathic pathogenetic trials**) who share common characteristics may be particularly sensitive to the effects of particular substances. Similarly some patients of common constitutional type respond well to particular homeopathic medicines.

5 In some traditions the concept of constitution takes on a different meaning, based mainly on **morphology**. Here, psychological and physiological characteristics and illness tendencies have marginal importance in the makeup of the constitution.

See also: **constitutional medicine, constitutional prescribing, carbonic constitution, epidemic constitution, fluoric constitution, Nebel, phosphoric constitution, sensitive type, sulphuric constitution, susceptibility, typology**

Etymology: L *com, cum* with + *statuere* to set up

constitutional medicine

● Medical methods, Therapeutics

1 System of homeopathy based on three constitutions described by Eduard von **Grauvogl** in 1865.

2 Grauvogl sought to relate the variation of patients' symptoms to their 'biochemical states' and their reaction to climate. He described three constitutions which appeared to follow the changes that took place in the blood and respiration. These were oxygenoid, hydrogenoid and carbo-nitrogenoid which some writers have said correspond to Hahnemann's three miasms. Grauvogl ascribed certain remedies to each constitution.

Comment:

1 This theory may have influenced **Schüssler** in his development of the **tissue salts**.

2 Grauvogl's classification was later superseded by the morphological–constitutional classification of types (**carbonic**, **fluoric** and **phosphoric**) by **Nebel**.

See also: **constitution, constitutional prescribing, morphology, typology**

constitutional prescribing

● Therapeutics

Choice of homeopathic prescription based on the study of the patient's **constitution** rather than the **clinical picture** alone.

See also: **clinical picture, constitution, constitutional medicine, morphology, similimum, typology**

constitutional remedy

● Therapeutics

Homeopathic medicine which matches patient's **constitution**.

See also: **constitutional prescribing**

consultation

● Therapeutics

1 The process of deliberating upon, or seeking information or advice about a subject, usually with another person.

2 The encounter and interaction between patient and practitioner for the purpose of diagnosis, prognosis or treatment, or to assess the progress of a **disease** or **illness**; may involve examination and simple investigation.

3 A meeting between two or more practitioners for the same purpose.

See also: **therapeutic encounter**

Etymology: L *consulere* to take counsel

continuous fluxion

See: **fluxion**

contradictory modality

● Materia medica, Symptomatology

A local **modality** (modality of a **local symptom**) which contradicts the general state of the patient. Some homeopathic medicines exhibit such modalities. For example, the **amelioration** of local symptoms by cold applications in a patient who is generally intolerant of the cold is a characteristic of *Ledum palustre*.

contraria contrariis curentur

● History, Philosophy

Latin phrase meaning 'Let contrary things be cured by contrary things'. It expresses the principle of **antipathic medicine**.

See also: **similia principle, similia similibus curentur**

control

● Research

1 To exert control over; to regulate, check or verify; in

research, to manage or take into account extraneous influences.

2 A standard of comparison used to check the results of an experiment. In a clinical experiment to evaluate a medical intervention, a subject or subjects receiving no intervention, or an alternative intervention (including **placebo**), who may be another patient or group of patients, or the same patient at different times. A different part of the same patient's body may also be used as a control.

See also: **blinding, homeopathic pathogenetic trial, randomised controlled trial**

controlled clinical trial

See: **randomised controlled trial**

conventional medicine

● Medical methods

The prevailing precepts and practice of contemporary western medicine. Otherwise known as **orthodox** or mainstream medicine.

Comment:
It is obviously true that other methods of medical practice may be conventional within the culture in which they are applied. The term 'conventional' is appropriated to contemporary western medicine because of its dominance of healthcare ideology. The boundaries of what is conventional are not fixed, however, but constantly changing.

See also: **allopathy, medical model, orthodox**
Etymology : L *cum* with + *venire* to come

correspondence

See: **similia principle**

cost-benefit analysis, cost-effectiveness analysis, cost-minimisation analysis, cost-utility analysis

See: **economic evaluation**

counteraction

● Philosophy

The automatic reaction of the **life force** to the initial action (**primary action**) of the homeopathic medicine. Also known as the **secondary drug action**.

Synonyms: **after action, back action**

creams

See: **dosage form**

crude material, crude substance

See: **source material**

crystal

● Pharmacy

1 A solid of regular shape in which the molecules are arranged in distinctive symmetrical patterns and, for a given compound, with its faces at characteristic angles; formed by freezing or precipitation when an element or chemical compound solidifies slowly enough for the individual molecules to take up regular positions with respect to one another.

2 In homeopathic pharmacy, a solid **dosage form** with the appearance of domestic granulated sugar and composed of **sucrose**.

Cullen, William

● History

Highly esteemed and influential Scottish physician (1710–1790). Regarded the nervous system (though he did not comprehend it in any sense as we do today) rather than the vascular system as the seat of all diseases, which he regarded as being provoked by environmental stimuli. He developed an early **nosology** consisting of four classes, based on the traditional physiological functions, animal, vital and natural, and also local pathological changes. These were respectively pyrexias, neuroses, cachexias and local disease.

Cullen lectured in many disciplines in medicine and the natural sciences, including **materia medica**. While Hahnemann was translating Cullen's *Treatise on Materia Medica* in 1790 he disagreed with his explanation of the action of Peruvian bark (cinchona) in intermittent or marsh fever (malaria). He took the medicine himself and found that he developed the symptoms of the fever. The realisation that a medicine that caused symptoms could cure them led him to formulate the **similia principle**.

See also: **cinchona**

cure

● Healing processes, Philosophy, Therapeutics

1   To eradicate **disease**; restore to **health**.
2   The removal or resolution of the symptoms, the **illness** or the disease process.
3   The means of achieving these aims. The **remedy**.

Comment:
The concept of cure in homeopathy is **holistic**. The eradication of a particular pathological process or syndrome is not the sole criterion of successful outcome. Change for the better in all aspects of the health and wellbeing of the patient is the ideal.

See also: **direction of cure, healing**
Etymology: L *curare* to take care of (*cura* care)

cyclical remedies

● Materia medica, Therapeutics

A group of homeopathic medicines which often seem to be indicated one after another in a cyclical fashion in a particular patient. For example, *Sulphur–Calcarea carbonica–Lycopodium*.

See also: **following remedy, relationship of remedies**

d

D potency

Abbreviation for: **decimal potency** (also written as x potency)

decimal potency

● Pharmacy, Therapeutics

1 A dilution in the proportion of 1 part in 10.
2 The sequential addition of 1 part of the **stock** or of the previous solution to 9 parts of **diluent**. The number of **serial dilutions** performed in this manner, with **succussion**, defines the decimal potency.

Comment:
The potencies are designated by a number with the letter 'x' following it. Thus 6x represents a 1 in 10 dilution carried out serially 6 times, with succussion at each stage. In some countries the x is replaced by

Dilution	Concentration	Decimal potency
1/10	10^{-1}	1x or D1
1/100	10^{-2}	2x or D2
1/1000	10^{-3}	3x or D3
1/10 000	10^{-4}	4x or D4
1/100 000	10^{-5}	5x or D5
1/1000 000	10^{-6}	6x or D6
$1/10^{30}$	10^{-30}	30x or D30

a letter D before the number signifying the number of dilutions (e.g. Euphrasia D6 is equivalent to Euphrasia 6x). Examples of decimal potencies are given on page 7:

Synonym: **D potency, DH potency, x potency**

See also: **centesimal potency, Hahnemannian potency, Korsakov potency, LM potency, millesimal potency, serial dilution**

Etymology: L *decimus* tenth (*decem* ten)

defective case

See: **one-sided case**

desensitisation

● Medical methods

Eliminating or neutralising the tendency to **hypersensitivity** and **allergy**. The usual method is exposure to very small but gradually increasing doses of the **allergen** (the provocative substance) until the immune system achieves tolerance of it.

Comment:
Various prescribing strategies in homeopathy are aimed at achieving this outcome. The one most easily compared to conventional desensitisation is the use of **isopathy**, though the physiological mechanism may be quite different.

desire

● Symptomatology

Thing or state for which the patient longs. Desire exceeds mere liking and may indicate a disturbance of the patient's equilibrium. At its most extreme amounts to a craving. Relates to foods, environmental factors, circumstances and situations, activities, psychological needs (e.g. desire for approval); any factor which affects the physical or emotional comfort of the individual. Such factors may be an important feature of the **constitution** or **clinical picture**.

See also: **aversion**

destruction of potency

● Biophysics and biochemistry, Pharmacology and drug action

Destruction of the active property of homeopathic medicines. It may be complete or partial and caused by biological, chemical, environmental or physical action.

Comment:

1 Certain conditions are essential to the preservation and transmission of potency **information**. If they are not present or are interfered with the active property of the preparation will be destroyed. Conditions that destroy potency are said to include the wrong chemical constituents of the diluent (polar diluents are believed to be necessary), interference with these constituents, heating, freezing, X-ray, microwave, ultrasound and electromagnetic fields. It is believed that these factors may be destructive of potency during storage or administration of the medicine. At present there is no definite experimental confirmation.

2 In practice patients are often warned to avoid handling the medicine, taking medicines too soon before or after food and drink, and exposing them to aromatic substances, but there is no evidence to confirm the deleterious effects of these.

Synonym: **inhibition of potency**
See also: **antidote, stability of drug**

destructive diathesis

See: **syphilitic miasm**

DH potency

See: **decimal potency, D potency, x potency**

Dhawale, M L

● Biography

Leading Indian homeopathic doctor (1927–1987).

Author of *Principles and Practice of Homoeopathy.*
He established the Clinical Research Institute in
Bombay.

d'Hervilly, Melanie

See: **Hahnemann, Melanie**

diadote

● Pharmacology and drug action, Therapeutics

An **antidote** to the action of homeopathic medicines
which is thought to interfere with their absorption by
its vasoconstrictor activity.

Etymology: GK *dia* through, apart + *doton* given

diagnosis

● Case taking and analysis

1 The process of formulating and formalising the
nature of the clinical problem through
enquiry, observation, examination and
investigation.

2 A formal statement of the clinical problem so derived
which integrates the various data.

3 Judgement or decision on the nature of the disease
process.

4 In homeopathic prescribing, the process of
determining the correct prescription.

Comment:
In conventional medicine the diagnosis is not
necessarily a statement of the underlying pathological
disorder. It is sometimes expressed in symptomatic
terms when no disease has been identified, or as an
interpretation of the problem in psychological or
social terms. Similarly, the **homeopathic diagnosis**
may represent the interpretation of the problem in
terms of the **drug picture** that corresponds to the
clinical picture.

Etymology: Gk *dia* through + *gignoskein* perceive,
recognise

diathesis

- Case taking and analysis, Disease processes
1   Individual hereditary or acquired disposition to
    contract a particular type of disorder.
2   Pattern of disorder characteristic of an underlying
    disease trait which may be inherited or acquired (e.g.
    tubercular diathesis). Not necessarily indicative of the
    presence of the disease in the individual.
3   The inherited or acquired organic weakness and
    systemic inferiority which leads to the morbid
    disposition and specific pathological processes in the
    evolution of a disease (Koehler 1986).

   Comment:
   Particular schools of homeopathy distinguish
   lymphatic diathesis (**psora**; **lymphatism**), **tubercular
   diathesis** (**pseudo-psora**), sycotic diathesis (**sycosis**)
   and syphilitic diathesis (**syphilis** = luetic diathesis =
   destructive diathesis) which are closely related to the
   concept of **miasm**.
   See also: **constitution, psora, sycosis, syphilis,
   terrain, tubercular diathesis**
   Etymology: Gk *dia* through + *tithemai* to arrange.

differential diagnosis

- Case taking and analysis, Disease processes, Therapeutics
1   The process of determining which of a number of
    disorders with similar clinical characteristics is
    actually affecting the patient; a comparative analysis of
    the possible **diagnoses**.
2   In homeopathy, the concept is also applied to the
    choice between a number of medicines whose **drug
    picture** shows some correspondence to the **clinical
    picture** in the patient.
   See also: **homeopathic diagnosis**

diluent

- Biophysics and biochemistry, Pharmacy
1   Substance used to achieve **dilution**; diluting agent.

2   In pharmacy generally, a substance used to achieve dilution which has no pharmacological activity of its own.

3   In homeopathy, the substance to which source material, the **stock** or a previous **potency** of the source material is added to dilute it for **potentisation**. Distilled or purified water, ethanol, ethanol–water mixtures, glycerine 85% or isotonic sodium chloride solution are used for liquids and soluble substances, lactose for **trituration** of insoluble substances. In the preparation of a **Hahnemannian potency** the diluent is deionised water and pharmaceutical alcohol in a concentration of 20% to 60%.

Etymology: L *diluere* f. *di-* through, apart + *luere* wash

dilution

- Pharmacy

1   Reduction in **concentration**, strength or quality of a substance by adding some other substance to it; usually the addition of water or some other liquid. The product of this process.

2   A stage in the preparation of a homeopathic medicine from its **stock** or previous **potency** by adding one part to a prescribed number of parts of **diluent** prior to **succussion**.

Comment:

1   For an illustration of different scales of dilution see **potency scales**.

2   Although the usual sense of the term refers to liquid dilution, in homeopathy early stages of dilution may be achieved by **trituration** using **lactose** as the diluent.

3   There are various methods of performing the liquid stages of dilution, for which see **fluxion, Hahnemannian potency, Korsakov potency, multiglass method, single glass method**.

See also: **attenuation, potentisation, ultrahigh dilution, ultramolecular dilution**

Etymology: L *diluere* f. *di-* through, apart + *luere* wash

direction of cure

● Case taking and analysis, Healing processes, Therapeutics

Criteria of healing change. Progressive improvement in the patient's state is indicated by changes in the disease process which have the following 'directions':

◆ from above downwards: symptoms progress and recede in a downward direction;
◆ from within outwards: from more deep-seated to more superficial organs;
◆ from the mental level to the physical level and from more important to less important organs;
◆ from most recent to previously occurring symptoms: symptoms resolve in reverse order of their onset.

Thus increase in certain symptoms may be indicative of good progress, if they are accompanied by other changes in a positive 'direction'. For example, in an atopic patient increase in eczema accompanying resolution of asthma is following the 'direction of cure'. Similarly, progress in a negative direction, even when there is improvement in a presenting symptom, indicates an unfavourable outcome of treatment.

The 'law' of direction of cure is one of the so called **laws of cure**, attributed to **Hering**.

Synonym: **Hering's criteria, Hering's law, Hering's rule**

See also: **cure, evolution of the case, palliation, reappearance of old symptoms, suppression**

disease

● Disease processes, Philosophy

1 Disorder of the tissues, organs, or physiological systems of an organism, or their functions.
2 A particular disorder identified by some combination of a distinctive cause, characteristic (**pathognomonic**) **symptoms** or **signs**, or anatomical, cellular or biochemical abnormalities.

Comment:

1 The concept of disease may include conditions in which the symptoms do not arise from an objectively identifiable disorder such as described above. Such conditions may better be described as **illness**, rather than disease. The concept of illness is more individual and subjective, lacking the objective, tangible or measurable characteristics of disease.

2 Similarly, disease processes, such as hypertension, may exist in the absence of any subjective disorder or distress.

3 The concept of disease in homeopathy has a wider meaning than in conventional thought. It encompasses the whole **clinical picture**, sometimes called the **disease picture**, rather than focusing on a particular pathological entity, diagnosis or syndrome. **Hahnemann** regarded disease as comprising all the perceptible symptoms and signs of disorder felt by the patient, perceived by those around him or observed by the physician. He attributed it to a derangement of the **life force**, but recognised the role of external factors in the causation of disease, including environmental factors, and he anticipated the discovery of the role of microorganisms in disease.

See also: **health**

Etymology: OF *desaise* without ease

disease affinity

● Materia Medica, Therapeutics

Some homeopathic medicines are particularly associated with specific pathological processes or diseases that occur prominently in their materia medica. For example, bruising and damage to small blood vessels are traditionally associated with *Arnica montana*. This is *Arnica*'s disease affinity.

Synonym: **pathotropism**

See also: **etiological prescribing, affinities, elective affinity, organ affinity, tissue affinity**

disease picture

● Case taking and analysis

Description of all the features of the **disease** in the individual patient. Virtually synonymous with **clinical picture**, but may imply emphasis on physical and pathological features.

See also: **drug picture, picture, symptom picture, totality of symptoms**

disease process

● Disease processes, Pathology
1 The **nosology** and **phenomenology** of disease.
2 The development and behaviour of a disease. Its effects in the mind or body.

See also: **evolution, pathography**

disorder

● Disease processes, Pathology, Symptomatology

An abnormal or disturbed state of mind or body.

disposition

● Constitution, morphology and terrain
1 Arrangement.
2 Tendency towards a certain state; natural tendency.

See also: **constitution, terrain, trait**

doctor

● Practitioner
1 One who has achieved a doctoral thesis.
2 **Physician**; graduate of a medical school.

See also: **clinician, lay homeopath, non-medically-qualified practitioner, physician, professional homeopath**

Etymology: L *docere* to teach

doctor–patient relationship

● Case taking and analysis, Therapeutics

Dynamics of practitioner–patient interaction; of the

therapeutic encounter. In homeopathy, in common with all **clinical** practice, this is the cornerstone of good **case taking** and **therapeutics**.

doctrine

● Philosophy, Therapeutics

1   The belief or system of instruction which is taught.
2   Philosophy or main principles upon which the teaching and practice of a particular system of medicine (e.g. homeopathy) is based; may be associated with a particular school or pattern of practice.
   Etymology: L *doctrina* teaching

doctrine of signatures

See: **signatures, doctrine of**

dosage form

● Pharmacy, Therapeutics

The form in which a medicine is presented for **administration**. The most common variants are listed in Box.
Synonym: **presentation**
See also: **dosage regime, dose, posology**

Solid dose forms

In conventional pharmacy tablets and capsules are made in different forms to control the speed at which the active ingredient is delivered. In homeopathy we are not faced with this necessity, so the choice of 'carrier' is governed by convenience rather than therapeutic efficiency. There is presently no standard for solid dose forms in the **pharmacopeias**, so size and ingredients vary from one manufacturer to another.

→

→

Tablets are similar to the classical biconvex plain white product used widely in conventional medicine. They are manufactured from **lactose** with **sucrose** and other appropriate **excipients**.

Pills, Pillules, Globules are spherical, like little balls. They are principally made from sucrose, layers of which are built up by adding aliquots of syrup to a seed granule in a revolving pan. Typical sizes are 2 mm (56 pills weigh 2 g) or 4 mm (56 pills weigh 4 g).

Globuli – see **Granules**

Granules are freeflowing sucrose granules that have the appearance of miniature **pillules**. Fine and coarse variants exist. May also be called **globuli** although these tend to comprise rather larger particles. There do not appear to be standards attached to the use of granules or globuli. The German Homeopathic Pharmacopeia does not make any distinction between the two. They are particularly useful for infants and animals. Dose is often written as 'sufficient granules to cover the cap liner of the bottle', 'give a pinch' or the amount required: '10 granules to be taken'.

Crystals are made of sucrose, and have the appearance of granulated sugar. They dissolve in water quickly and are good for infants as they tend to stick to the tongue better than granules. With the increasing preference for sugar-free medicines, crystals are declining in popularity.

Individual powders are especially useful for combined medicated and placebo treatments or where one remedy must follow another in sequence. Usually made from lactose impregnated with liquid **potency**, but crystals may also be used. The powders can be individually numbered in the correct sequence and the patient instructed to take the powders in order. Bulk powders have a pure lactose base. →

→

Liquids for oral administration

Occasionally **mother tinctures** may be given orally (e.g. *Crataegus*), usually in water. Liquid **potencies** prepared from the mother tinctures by **serial dilution** may also be given by mouth directly, in water or on a sugar cube. They are especially useful in veterinary applications when animals can be dosed effectively by adding the remedy to the drinking water. Both liquid potencies and mother tinctures may be incorporated in syrups, such as *Bryonia* cough mixture.

Topical products

Generic and speciality ointments, creams, lotions, oils and liniments contain varying percentages of a **mother tincture** (5–10%), or in a few cases liquid potency (e.g. *Graphites*, *Sulphur*), or triturations incorporated in a suitable **vehicle**. Homeopathic ointments are emollient preparations in an appropriate base (often lanolin–alcohol ointment or soft paraffin). Topical liquid preparations are prepared using ethanol–water mixtures or vegetable oil. Groundnut oil, olive oil and sesame oil are normally used. Glycerine may be used as an additive.

Other dosage forms

Eyedrops, such as those containing *Calendula* (minor infections), *Cineraria* (certain corneal opacities) and particularly *Euphrasia* (allergies) are available.

   Injections are especially popular on the continent of Europe and in the USA. For example, potencies of medicines such as *Ruta* and *Apis mellifica* are injected directly into painful muscles and periarticular tissues respectively.

→

→

Nasal sprays offer a convenient route of
administration.

Inhalation. A rare dosage form consists of a
small glass vial containing granules (globuli)
whose vapour is inhaled via the nose.

Suppositories of a homeopathic medicine in a
hard fat base may be used.

---

dosage regime

● Pharmacy, Therapeutics

1   Schedule of drug administration.

2   The complete specification of the amount and
frequency of the dose, or the schedule according to
which repeated or successive doses of the same or
other medicines are to be administered.

See also: **dosage form, dose, posology, repetition of
dose**

dose

● Pharmacy, Therapeutics

The amount of a medicine to be taken or administered
to a patient at any one time or in separate fractional
amounts over a given period.

Comment:

In homeopathy the dose should be the smallest
possible to bring about a therapeutic effect. Thus a
pinch of granules or one tablet or pill is sufficient as
a dose. Although today the quantity of a dose is
regarded by most practitioners as of little importance,
Hahnemann prescribed definite quantities.

Etymology: Gk. *dosis* giving, gift (*didonai* give)

See also: **dosage form, dosage regime, posology,
repetition of dose**

dose-dependent reverse effect

● Biophysics and biochemistry, Pharmacology and drug
action

The phenomenon in which different **doses** of a substance may produce opposite effects in a biological system.

See also: **antitaxic drug action, Arndt-Schulz law, biphasic activity, hormesis, primary drug action, secondary drug action**

dose repetition

See: **repetition of dose**

dose response curve

● Biophysics and biochemistry, Pharmacology and drug action

1 Variation in response relative to **dose**.
2 The graphical representation of the variation in response of a biological system in relation to the dose of an applied stimulus, usually pharmacological. For example, the graphical representation of **biphasic activity**.

See also: **Arndt-Schulz law, dose-dependent reverse effect, hormesis**

drainage therapy

● Medical methods, Therapeutics

The elimination of **toxins** believed to arise from the **disease process**, from physiological dysfunction or from the environment, which may have a debilitating or detrimental effect on the organism, before or during the individualised homeopathic regime. Drainage uses homeopathic medicines in **low potency** in frequent doses over a period of days or weeks. The medicine is chosen by reference to the organ system identified as needing the stimulus of drainage and the circumscribed symptoms shown by the patient relating to that system. Based on the hypothesis that there are organ-related toxins which will be eliminated thereby. The method was originally conceived in France and is used also in Germany.

See also: **antihomotoxic therapy, organ affinity, organotherapy**

drug

● Pharmacology and drug action, Pharmacy

1 Substance, other than a food or nutrient, capable of
  affecting physiological processes and influencing the
  functional or subjective state of the individual.
2 Pharmacologically active therapeutic agent.

Comment:
The term 'drug' is not commonly used in homeopathy
to describe the medicinal agent. **Homeopathic remedy**
or 'medicine' are the usual forms. The preferred term
'medicine' has been chosen for this dictionary, a usage
that is consistent with the editorial policy of the
British Homoeopathic Journal.
See also: **remedy**

drug action

● Pharmacology and drug action

The effect of a drug on the biological system as
distinct from its activity at a biochemical level.

Comment:
The difference between homeopathic and conventional
drug action may be said to be that whereas the latter
generally acts to control or manipulate body function
or disease processes, homeopathic medicines have
claimed to enable or reinforce natural self-regulatory
processes. Replacement therapies are an exception to
this distinction.
See also: **autoregulation**

drug interaction

● Pharmacology and drug action, Therapeutics

The influence, desirable or undesirable, of one **drug**
upon another; may be **synergistic**, reinforcing,
inimical or **antidotal**. Interactions may also involve
physiologically-occurring chemical substances,
chemicals in the diet or chemicals introduced to the
body for other purposes such as investigations.

Comment:
Although homeopathic medicines may be used in a complementary manner, as when a **bowel nosode** is used to support the action of one of the medicines associated with it, they are not believed to interact in the conventional sense.

See also: **antidote, compatible, inimical, synergism**

drug picture

● Case taking and analysis, Materia medica, Symptomatology, Therapeutics.

1 The characteristic clinical features of the **materia medica** of a homeopathic medicine; comprises all the recorded **mental**, **general** and **local** (particular) **symptoms** and signs, **modalities**, and pathological changes and test findings if appropriate.

2 Sometimes used to refer only to the main characteristic symptoms of the medicine.

Comment:

1 The main basis of the drug picture are the experimental symptoms obtained by **homeopathic pathogenetic trials** (**provings**). These, together with clinically verified symptoms cured after administration of the medicine to sick people, and toxicological symptoms observed after poisonous doses, build up the symptom complex unique to each medicine. Thus the drug picture is a detailed collection of all the effects which the medicine can cause in human beings. This comprehensive compilation explains the wide range of medicinal effects given for each homeopathic medicine.

2 The drug pictures written by **Kent** and particularly by **Tyler** used a descriptive form which made the **materia medica** easy to remember. They had the disadvantage of sometimes presenting a picture from which variation of symptomatology was omitted, and of being coloured by the social and cultural context of the author's practice.

Synonym: **remedy picture**

See also: **case analysis, case taking, clinical picture, disease picture, guiding symptoms, keynotes, materia medica, pathogenesis**

drug type

See: **typology**

Dudgeon, Robert Ellis

● Biography

British physician (1820–1904), of the rationalist school. He was co-editor of the *British Journal of Homoeopathy* from 1846 until it closed in 1884. He wrote many articles on homeopathy and homeopathic tracts. His translations from **Hahnemann** include the fifth edition of the **Organon** in 1849, ***Materia Medica Pura*** in 1880 and *Lesser Writings* in 1851. He served as Secretary of the English Homoeopathic Association and helped in the foundation of the Hahnemann Hospital, London, where he gave his **Lectures on the Theory and Practice of Homoeopathy**. While loyal to the **similia principle**, he criticised Hahnemann's theories. He was one of the last medical generalists, inventing spectacles for use under water, modifying Marey's sphygmograph for clinical use, and writing a book on the prolongation of life. He refused to accept **Kent**'s ideas on **constitutional prescribing** which arrived in Britain shortly before his own death.

dynamis

● Philosophy

Hahnemann's term for the spirit-like force (**life force**) that animates the material organism.

See also: **bioenergetics, dynamisation, life force, potency, potency energy, potentisation, vital force, Wesen**

Etymology: Gk *dunamis* power

dynamisation

● Biophysics and biochemistry, Pharmacology and drug action, Pharmacy

The process by which the therapeutic activity or medicinal power of a homeopathic medicine is released or enhanced. This is achieved initially by **trituration** for insoluble substances and by **serial dilution** and **succussion** for soluble substances and those rendered soluble after trituration. Also known as **potentisation**, which see for discussion of the ambiguity in the use of the two terms. Succussion is essential to this process. Dilution alone is not effective.

See also: **attenuation, dynamis, plussing**

eclectic

- Philosophy

  Embracing a variety of ideas and methods; not exclusive; not committed to one particular **doctrine**.

  Etymology: Gk *eklectikos* selective (*ek-* out + *legein* choose)

eclectic colleges

- History

  Medical schools in the USA in the 19th century, claiming to teach the best of all systems of medicine, principally **phytotherapy**, also homeopathy and elements of native American medicine, and eschewing the more drastic therapies such as bleeding and purging which were prevalent at the time. Some of the eclectic colleges were of a poor standard, and most of them were closed after the publication of the **Flexner Report**.

eclectic medicine

- Medical methods, Philosophy, Therapeutics
1 System of medicine employing a variety of therapeutic methods; **eclectic**.
2 Therapeutic method in which a combination of homeopathic medicines (complex or single remedies), **phytotherapy** and **allopathic** medicines may be

prescribed. It existed as a formal system in the US in the late 19th century.

Comment:
This is not an **orthodox** homeopathic method, but it can be useful in specific cases.

See also: **complex homeopathy, eclectic colleges, Kent, pluralist homeopathy, unicist homeopathy**

Etymology: Gk eklectikos selective (ek- out + legein choose)

economic evaluation

● Research

Systematic identification, measurement and where appropriate, valuation of all the relevant costs and consequences of the options under review.

Comment:
An increasingly important aspect of the evaluation of homeopathic medicines. Different kinds of analysis are:

◆ **cost-benefit analysis** economic evaluation involving estimate of monetary value of benefits or outcomes of interventions. Analysis includes direct costs of treatment, but also indirect costs such as time lost from work and social security payments as well as broader social and economic costs to society as a whole.

◆ **cost-effectiveness analysis** economic evaluation involving analysis of costs of interventions when outcomes of interventions may vary, but can be expressed in common natural units.

◆ **cost-minimisation analysis** economic evaluation involving analysis of costs where the outcomes of procedures are the same or similar.

◆ **cost-utility analysis** economic evaluation comparing interventions in different diseases where outcomes have no common standard of measurement. Utility refers to subjective satisfaction and may be measured in terms of units such as Quality Adjusted Life Years (QALYs).

Etymology: Gk *oikonomos* steward (*oikos* house + *-nomos* f. *nemo* manage)

effectiveness

● Research

The extent to which a specific intervention, procedure or regime does what it is intended to do for a specified population, when deployed in the field in routine circumstances.

efficacy

● Research

The extent to which a specific intervention, procedure or regime does what it is intended to do for a specified population, when applied in ideal circumstances.

elective affinity

● Materia medica, Therapeutics

The anatomical structure or body system that is the particular seat of action of a homeopathic medicine.

See also: **disease affinity, organ affinity, tissue affinity**

Etymology: L *e- legere* pick

eliminating symptom

● Symptomatology, Therapeutics

A **symptom** of such importance that it is used to simplify the choice of homeopathic prescription by excluding those medicines in whose **materia medica** it does not appear.

See also: **elimination**

Etymology: L *e- +liminare* (*limen* threshold)

elimination

● Physiology, Symptomatology, Therapeutics

1 The process by which something is removed or got rid of.

2   The process by which the body rids itself of waste and
    toxic substances by secretion or excretion.
3   The phenomenon of increase in secretions or
    excretory functions, or the appearance of a skin
    eruption, in response to homeopathic treatment.
4   The process by which the choice of the homeopathic
    prescription is simplified by excluding those
    medicines which do not have a chosen **eliminating**
    symptom in their **materia medica**.
    Etymology: L e- +*liminare* (*limen* threshold)

emanometer

> *See:* **Boyd, William Ernest**

emotion

● Symptomatology

1   A mental state concerned with feeling rather than
    consciousness, reasoning and intellect; metaphorically
    associated with the heart.
2   A category of **mental symptom**.
    Synonym: **affect**

empirical

● Philosophy, Research

Deriving knowledge from experience or observation,
rather than on the basis of theory.

Comment:
The scientific origins of homeopathy were essentially
empirical. Most of its knowledge base is derived from
observation in the first instance. A scientific weakness
in homeopathy is to rest on the empirical justification
for its principles without resolving these into testable
hypotheses.
See also: **empirical medicine**
Etymology: Gk *empeirikos* (*empeiria* experience f.
empeiros skilled)

empirical medicine

● History, Medical methods

Practice of medicine founded on experience alone, rather than on reasoning or theory, deduction or investigation.

Etymology: Gk *empeirikos* (*empeiria* experience f. *empeiros* skilled)

enantiopathic

See: **antipathic**

Etymology: Gk *enantios* opposite + *patheia* suffering

endemic

● Disease processes

Occurring regularly or only found within a particular population or geographical area. For example, typhoid and **malaria** are endemic to certain parts of the world.

Etymology: Gk *endemos* native (*demos* people)

energy

● Philosophy, Physiology, Therapeutics

1 Vigour, **vitality**.
2 The ability to do work or to produce an effect.

Comment:

In homeopathy the patient's energy or vitality, and changes in energy and vitality are important in assessing his or her well-being, capacity to respond to and actual response to treatment.

See also: **biodynamics, bioenergetics, dynamis, life force**

Etymology: Gk *en-* +*ergon* work

entelechy

● Philosophy

The complete realisation of potential; the full expression of the properties or qualities inherent in a system. Principle expounded by Aristotle (c.384–322 BCE).

Comment:
Fundamental principle of **holism**. The action of homeopathic medicines is believed to promote entelechy.
Etymology: Gk *en telei ekho* to be in perfection.

environment

● Case taking and analysis, Disease processes, Healing processes

Surroundings, conditions, circumstances of existence.
Etymology: OF *environ* (*en* in + *viron* circuit f. *virer* to turn)

environmental factors

● Case taking and analysis, Disease processes, Healing processes, Symptomatology

Factors in the **environment** which influence events, particularly in relation to health or wellbeing. Such factors are important in understanding the etiology of some illnesses, an individual's reactions and behaviour and the behaviour of symptoms, and are of particular significance in homeopathic therapeutics.
See also: **aversion, desire, general symptom, modality, temperature modality, weather modality**

epidemic

● Disease processes

1 **Disease** or **illness** that affects many people at the same time, usually by the same **causative** agent.
2 Widespread outbreak of a disease within a community, population or region; also used to describe outbreaks of disease in animals or plants.
See also: **endemic**
Etymology: Gk *epi* upon + *demos* the people

epidemic constitution

● Disease processes

Characteristics of people that make them susceptible to **epidemic** diseases.

Comment:
The epidemic constitution was identified by Thomas **Sydenham** (1624–1689). It anticipates to an extent the homeopathic concepts of **constitution**, **terrain** and **typology**.

epidemic diseases

⬤ History

It was the success of homeopathy in treating **epidemic** diseases such as **cholera**, **scarlet fever** and **typhus** that first demonstrated its **effectiveness**.

epidemic remedy

⬤ Therapeutics

Homeopathic medicine that has proved curative in an **epidemic** disease. Homeopathic medicine whose **drug picture** corresponds to the **disease picture** of a particular **epidemic**.

Comment:
Victims of the same **epidemic** disease usually show a similar **clinical picture**. The appropriate **simillimum** may be used to treat all sufferers from that epidemic. An example is the use of *Belladonna* in **scarlet fever**.

Synonym: **genus epidemicus**
See also: **disease affinity**

essence

⬤ Case taking and analysis, Materia medica

1 All that makes a thing what it is; intrinsic nature.
2 In homeopathy the unique character of a medicine's **materia medica**; its **individuality**; usually expressed in psychological or abstract terms which often reflect metaphorically the physical characteristics.

Synonym: **genius of the remedy**
See also: **Wesen**
Etymology: L *esse* to be

etiology

● Disease processes

1 The study of **causality**; the attribution of cause.
2 The study of the causes of **disease.**
3 The attribution of the cause of the **illness**.

Comment:
Homeopathy places particular emphasis on etiology, not only for understanding the patient and the illness, but also for choosing the prescription and determining the **prescribing strategy**. The concept of etiology is broader in **homeopathy** than in **conventional medicine** in this context, embracing a wider range of influences affecting the **evolution** and **onset of illness**, including psychological, social, physical and environmental factors.
See also: **ailments from, causal, causation, etiological prescribing, never well since, precipitating factor**
Etymology: Gk *aitiologia* study of cause (*aitia* cause)

etiological factor

● Disease processes

Any event or circumstance, medical or biographical, in the personal or family history of the patient which has been a cause of the illness.
See also: **ailments from, causal, causality, causation, never well since, precipitating factor**
Etymology: Gk *aitiologia* study of cause (*aitia* cause)

etiological prescribing

● Therapeutics

Homeopathic prescription based on **etiology**.
See also: **etiotropism, ailments from, isopathy, never well since, nosode, precipitating factor**
Etymology: Gk *aitiologia* study of cause (*aitia* cause)

etiotropism

● Materia medica, Therapeutics

Association of a homeopathic medicine with a particular **etiology**.

See also: **etiological prescribing**

Etymology: Gk *aitia* cause + *tropikos* turning

evaluation of symptoms

● Case taking and analysis, Symptomatology

The evaluation of **symptoms** by the clinician for their significance as indications for the choice of the prescription.

Criteria by which the value of symptoms is judged include:

◆ the spontaneity and vividness with which they are presented;
◆ the degree of emphasis given to them by the patient;
◆ their individuality to the patient as compared to their common association with the disease process;
◆ the level at which they affect the patient, mental and emotional level being held to be of particular importance;
◆ their strangeness, rareness or peculiarity.

The process of evaluation is commonly represented by **weighting** the symptom (**ponderation**); representing the value of the symptom in the case notes by attributing a score (usually 1–4), or by underlining the symptom one or more times. The value of the symptom is taken into account in the **case analysis** and in **repertorisation**. Symptoms of greater value are emphasised when calculating the degree to which different medicines correspond to the **symptom picture**.

Synonyms: **grading of symptoms, ranking of symptoms**

See also: **case analysis, case taking, hierarchy of symptoms, symptom selection**

evidence

● Research

The data and the method by which they are obtained and analysed justifying a particular conclusion, or that establish a fact.

See also: **effectiveness, efficacy, empirical**

evidence-based medicine

● Medical methods, Research

Use of the best available and most valid evidence to make decisions about patient care, tempered by clinical judgement and experience.

Comment:
The elements of evidence-based medicine have been defined as: asking a focused question, finding the evidence, appraising the evidence, acting on the results, appraising one's own performance (Sackett and Rosenberg 1995). **Clinical trials** provide the most widely acceptable evidence, but observational and qualitative studies are also important, and certainly contribute to the evidence accepted by practising clinicians.

evolution

● Case taking and analysis, Disease processes, Healing processes

1   A process of gradual development, usually leading to a higher degree of organisation.
2   In homeopathy, the development of the patient's condition to its present state, seen in the context of the patient's life history, past and intercurrent medical history and response to the therapeutic intervention.

See also: **biopathography, pathogenesis**
Etymology: L *evolutio* unrolling (*volvere* to roll)

exacerbation

● Disease processes

1   Worsening of symptoms.
2   Increase in severity of the disease.

Comment:
The term exacerbation may be synonymous with **aggravation** in both conventional and homeopathic usage. In conventional use, however, it implies a change for the worse in the course of the disease, by contrast with the transient increase in symptoms in response to

the homeopathic prescription, which usually carries a good prognosis.

Etymology: L *ex-* bring into a state + *acerbus* bitter

excipient

⬢ Pharmacy

All the non-medicinal components of the **dosage form** (e.g. binders, preservatives.)

See also: **adjuvant, auxilliary substance, vehicle**

Etymology: L *excipiens* (*ex-* + *cipio* take out)

exciting cause

See: **etiology, onset, precipitating factor**

experiment

⬢ Research

1 A trial or test; to make trial of, to test.
2 Procedure undertaken on the chance that it may succeed.
3 Procedure undertaken to test a **hypothesis**.

Etymology: L *experimentum* (*ex-* + *periri* to try)

experimental pathogenesis

See: **homeopathic pathogenetic trial**

expressed juice

⬢ Pharmacy

The juices expressed from fresh plants, used to prepare a **mother tincture**. The juice is diluted with an equal part of 86% ethanol to precipitate the main part of the proteins and other insoluble compounds; after filtration the mother tincture is obtained.

external treatment

See: **dosage form, local treatment**

f

F

Abbreviation for: **fluxion**

family

● Materia medica, Therapeutics

1 A group that shares common ancestry.
2 A group that shares common characteristics by which it can be classified.
3 Members of the same household who share a common affiliation.
4 In homeopathy, the members of a particular class of homeopathic medicines. This may include biological families such as the snake medicines, derived from snake venom, or chemical relationships, as in the 'family' of *Calcium* salts.

See also: **theme**

fifty millesimal potency

See: **LM potency**

Flexner Report

● History

Report entitled *Medical Education in the United States and Canada* written by Abraham Flexner and published in 1910 for the Carnegie Foundation in cooperation with the American Medical Association.

The report insisted on the need for a thorough academic and scientific education as a basis for medical qualification, and severely criticised the low standards in most medical colleges. It proposed that the number of colleges should be reduced and their quality greatly improved. The result was that good graduates were precluded from registration because they trained at 'poor' schools. All homeopathic colleges were graded poor. The report contributed to the decline of homeopathy in North America in the early 1900s, and of 22 colleges of homeopathy existing in 1900 only seven remained by 1918. The last closed in the 1930s. Registerable homeopathic medical qualifications, therefore, disappeared. Postgraduate teaching for doctors by the American Foundation for Homeopathy began in 1922.

fluoric constitution

● Constitution, morphology and terrain

The association described by **Nebel** of angular or asymmetrical people, usually thin, possibly undernourished, and with lax ligaments and hyperextensible joints, with the characteristics of the homeopathic medicine *Calcarea fluorica*.

See also: **carbonic constitution, constitution, Grauvogl, morphology, phosphoric constitution, sulphuric constitution, typology**

fluxion

● Pharmacy

A method of manufacture of liquid **potencies** without **succussion** strokes. The potentising effect is produced by the turbulence of flowing or injected water. Fluxion **potentisation** was developed by Bernhard Fincke who took out a patent in 1869. It is a special type of the **single glass method** and suitable for simple potentising machines producing **high potencies**.

Comment:

1 The method is not officially included in most

national **pharmacopeias**, and is now considered unreliable, but is still in use in Brazil, Argentina and possibly Mexico, and is included in the Brazilian homeopathic pharmacopeia (2nd edn, 1997).

2 Thomas Skinner, a Scottish physician (1825–1906), devised the Skinner Continuous Fluxion Apparatus still used for the mechanical production of **millesimal potencies**.

Synonym: **continuous fluxion**

Etymology: L *fluere* to flow

following remedy

● Materia medica, Therapeutics

A medicine that follows well after the administration of another medicine. Named 'remedies that follow well' by Gibson **Miller**, 'follow well' by **Hering** or 'remedies following' by **Guernsey**.

See also: **compatible, concordances**

force

● Philosophy

1 An external influence which tends to produce motion in a body.

2 **Hahnemann**'s concept of the source of those changes and processes in the organism which cannot be perceived by the human senses.

See also: **dynamis**

Etymology: L *fortis* strong

Foubister, Donald

● Biography

Scottish physician (1902–1988). He worked at the Royal London Homoeopathic Hospital for many years, and was largely responsible for pioneering the use of *Carcinosin*.

frequently used remedies

● Materia medica, Therapeutics

Medicines which are frequently used, not necessarily

polychrests or major medicines.

See also: **major remedy, status of medicines**

fresh plant trituration

● Pharmacy

Alternative to the use of **mother tinctures** for the first steps in the process of **potentising** fresh plants. **Trituration** with **lactose** was recommended by **Hahnemann** in 1835 for all source materials including fresh plants and **expressed juice** because he found that the resulting medicines acted more powerfully and had a longer shelf life.

functional symptom

● Symptomatology

A symptom with no known or detectable organic basis.

Comment:

1 Based on our current knowledge, it is not easy to distinguish between functional and organic **symptoms**. The judgement is usually clinical and often subjective. But introduction of more sensitive diagnostic techniques has sometimes demonstrated that symptoms previously considered functional do have an organic basis.

2 Functional symptoms are given more significance as manifestations of disorder in homeopathy than is sometimes the case in **conventional medicine**.

See also: **symptom picture, totality of symptoms**

Etymology: L *functio* f. *fungi* perform

fundamental cause

● Disease processes

The deepest underlying cause of a disease, as distinct from the **occasion** or **precipitating factor**. For example, a **miasm**.

See also: **etiological factor, etiology, onset, pathogenesis**

g

Galen

● Biography, History

Roman physician of the second century AD, whose work exerted enormous influence on medical thought for many centuries. He was a pioneer anatomist, benefiting by an early appointment as physician to gladiators whose wounds afforded plenty of opportunity for such studies. He combined his experience of external and skeletal anatomy with philosophical speculation, to develop his system of medicine. This included a systematic account of concealed body structures and the importance of their functional integrity, and of the effect of deleterious 'humours' in the development of disease. He was a convinced advocate of the therapeutic value of bleeding in all cases, even loss of blood. His views on the circulation of the blood were accepted for many centuries, until disproved by Harvey (1578–1657).

gemmotherapy

● Medical methods

Use of fresh plant extracts in therapy; usually the embryonic parts such as buds and shoots.

See also: **herbal medicine**

Etymology: L *gemma* bud

general symptom

● Case taking and analysis, Symptomatology

1 Symptom that applies to the patient as a
  whole rather than to a specific part or system;
  the organism's overall response to the
  disorder.
2 A general **characteristic** or reaction of the patient
  to such factors as temperature, weather, the time of
  day and food (**desires** and **aversions**). Some
  authors include functions such as perspiration,
  sexual appetite and sleep among the general
  symptoms.

  See also: **aggravating factor, environmental factors,
  modality**

genius of the remedy

  See: **essence**

genus epidemicus

  See: **epidemic remedy**

grading of symptoms

  See: **evaluation of symptoms, repertorisation,
  rubric, weighting of symptoms**

grafting

● Pharmacy

1 The act of inserting or attaching one piece of
  living tissue to another to form a permanent union.
2 In homeopathy, the process of adding further
  unmedicated tablets (or another dosage form) to
  the remains of an existing supply of **potentised**
  medicine.

  Comment:
  This is not a recognised method in homeopathic
  pharmacy, is not represented in the pharmacopeias,
  and is deprecated by most practitioners.

Grauvogl, Eduard von

● Biography

German physician (1811–1877). He sought to relate the variation of patients' symptoms to their 'biochemical states' and their reaction to climate. He described three constitutions which appeared to follow the changes that took place in the blood and respiration. These were **oxygenoid**, **hydrogenoid** and **carbo-nitrogenoid** which some writers have said correspond to Hahnemann's three **miasms**. Grauvogl ascribed certain remedies to each **constitution**. His classification was later superseded by **Nebel**'s.

See also: **constitutional medicine, morphology, typology**

grinding

● Pharmacy

Method used in the preparation of homeopathic medicines from solid material by **trituration**. Involves grinding the solid, together with a suitable vehicle such as **lactose**, by hand with pestle and mortar or using a suitable machine.

Synonym: **pulverisation**

See also: **ball mill trituration**

group remedies

● Therapeutics

1 **Combination remedies** for specific conditions.
2 Medicines which can be studied as a group because they belong to a common **family** and share common characteristics.

See also: **complex homeopathy**

Guernsey, William Jefferson

● Biography

American physician (1854–1935). Professor of gynecology and later of **materia medica** in Philadelphia. He originated the **keynote** system.

guiding symptom

● Case taking and analysis, Materia medica, Symptomatology

Symptom that provides a strong indication for the choice of a particular medicine; symptom highly characteristic of a particular medicine.

Comment:
There is no clear distinction between guiding symptoms and **key note** symptoms. *Guiding Symptoms* was a **materia medica** written by **Hering** (1879) and described as a collection of cured symptoms, rather than those demonstrated solely by **provings**.

See also: **eliminating symptom**

h

Haehl, Richard

- Biography

Homeopathic practitioner in Stuttgart (1873–1923), he collected a vast number of documents relating to **Hahnemann**. With William **Boericke** he conducted negotiations with **Boenninghausen**'s family for 29 years before finally obtaining the manuscript of the sixth edition of the *Organon* which was published in 1921. He also wrote the authoritative *Samuel Hahnemann: His Life and Work*.

Hahnemann, Christian Friedrich Samuel

- Biography

Physician and founder of homeopathy (1755–1843). An expert linguist, while still adolescent he went to Vienna to study medicine. Short of money he took employment with the Governor of Transylvania. Here he became familiar with marsh fever (**malaria**). He finally qualified at Erlangen in 1779. He soon became disillusioned with the medicine of the time and increasingly occupied himself translating books into German. His disagreement with the ideas of William **Cullen** lead to his formulation of the **similia principle** which he published in 1796 as his *Essay on a New Principle*. The first edition of his definitive **Organon** followed in 1810. He invented a system of testing the action of medicines, which he called *Prüfung* (Ger for trial, anglicised as **proving**). His first results were published as *Fragmenta de Viribus* (1805), followed by *Materia Medica Pura* (1811–21). In 1812 he obtained permission to lecture at Leipzig University but his attacks upon the medical profession made him unpopular. Dispensing his own medicines brought him into conflict with the **apothecaries** who had the sole legal right to dispense. In 1819 they laid a complaint against him which was upheld. As a result he had to leave Leipzig for Köthen in 1821. He remained there until 1835, a semi-recluse, although in active practice. In 1829, he announced his theory of **chronic disease**, an explanation of why homeopathy sometimes failed. In 1835 he married Melanie **d'Hervilly** and moved to Paris, where he conducted a successful practice until his death.

Hahnemann, Melanie

● Biography

Married name of Marie Melanie d'Hervilly Gohier, Hahnemann's second wife (1800–1878). They married in 1835 and moved to Paris the following year. She was a poet and painter, and became a skilled homeopath, sharing in Hahnemann's practice in Paris and continuing to practise after his death. Melanie bore Hahnemann no children. She claimed unsuccessfully that a diploma from **Allentown Academy** entitled her to practise medicine in France, and was fined 100Ff for illegal practice. She jealously guarded the sixth edition of the *Organon* from publication.

Hahnemannian potency

● Pharmacy

Method originated by Samuel **Hahnemann** of performing the process of **serial dilution** in which one part taken from the preparation at the previous stage in the process is added to the requisite number of parts of **diluent** in a new glassware container at each stage (**multiglass method**) and submitted to **succussion**. The number of serial dilutions performed in this manner defines the **potency** according to the proportions used in the series. The method provides two scales of potency, **decimal** and **centesimal**.

Comment:
The German homeopathic pharmacopeia only permits the use of the Hahnemannian method for **potentisation**.

See also: **fluxion, korsakovian potency, LM potency, multiglass method, single glass method**

Hahnemannism

● History

Physical **force** described by **Hering** in support of the **dynamisation** theory. It was alleged that this homeopathic force allowed the communication by certain atoms of their character to other atoms, thus one potentised tablet could pass its **potency** to unmedicated tablets, and medicinal properties could be transferred to non-medicinal objects, so a bottle itself could be impregnated with a potency. The force could be insulated by cork and glass. The concept is not currently generally accepted by homeopaths.

See also: **grafting**

half homeopaths

● History

Pejorative term used by **Hahnemann** to describe those who mixed homeopathy with **allopathy**.

See also: **mongrel**

healing

● Healing processes, Philosophy, Therapeutics

Restoration of **health** or wholeness.

Comment:
1 Healing is distinct from **cure** and **treatment** because it involves a creative change in the

organism towards a state of greater wholeness; healing involves **entelechy**.

2 The concept of **cure** in homeopathy sometimes carries the meaning given here for healing, but this is not always the case, as when speaking of 'cured symptoms' in a more circumscribed sense.

Etymology: OE *hælan* to heal (*hal* whole)

healing crisis

● Disease processes, Healing processes

In conventional terms, the turning point of an illness which may be preceded by an intensification of symptoms, and is followed by rapid improvement. In homeopathy the term is sometimes used as a synonym to **therapeutic aggravation**.

health

● Philosophy, Therapeutics

1 The quality of soundness and wellbeing of an organism; soundness of mind and body.

2 The ability of the organism to retain its integrity while adapting to changing circumstances.

Comment:
Homeopathic thought regards health as a highly dynamic state, tending always towards optimum equilibrium by the operation of self-regulating, self-healing mechanisms. It is believed that homeopathic medicines act by stimulating these mechanisms. Wider definitions of health take account of the whole physical, psychological, social and spiritual wellbeing of the patient. This is certainly the homeopathic perspective of health.

See also: **autoregulation**

Etymology: OE *hælth* (*hal* whole)

healthy

● Philosophy, Therapeutics

In good **health**.

Henderson, William

● Biography

Professor of pathology at Edinburgh and pioneering microbiologist (1811–1872). He was ostracised when he converted to homeopathy in the 1840s and published his cases, was forced to resign from all the medical societies and only retained his professional chair because it was a lifetime appointment.

herbal medicine

● Medical methods

The medicinal use of plants, parts of plants or plant extracts.

Comment:

1 In Europe, herbal medicine shares a large number of common source materials with homeopathy, and in consequence the two are sometimes confused in popular perception.
2 Many different forms of herbal medicine exist in different parts of the world, reflecting differences in the local flora.

Synonyms: **herbalism, phytotherapy**

heredity

● Disease processes

1 The process of inheritance; the begetting of like by like.
2 Transmission of the characteristics or attributes of parents to their offspring. May be applied to social attributes such as wealth or status, but usually applied to biological characteristics transmitted by information, principally genetic, carried in the ovum and sperm.

Comment:

The concept of **miasm** includes the transmission of a hereditary **predisposition** to certain patterns of **disease**, but this is not necessarily associated with any known genetic mechanism.

See also: **constitution, disposition, predisposition, terrain, trait**

Etymology: L *hereditare* f. *heres* heir

Hering, Constantin

● Biography

German physician (1800–1880) who emigrated to America in 1833. As a medical student in Leipzig he attended **Hahnemann**'s lectures without being impressed with the merits of homeopathy. His tutor and Baumgarten, a publisher, suggested that he study the subject with a view to exposing its flaws. He was however converted and as a result had to move to Würzburg in order to qualify as a doctor. From 1827–1833 he was in Surinam where among other medicines he made a **proving** of *Lachesis*. After emigrating to America he was a co-founder of the **Allentown Academy** where all teaching was in German, but in 1848 he founded the Homeopathic Medical College of Philadelphia where English was the language used. In 1844 he was elected the first president of the **American Institute of Homeopathy**. He proved many remedies and published many papers. He also suggested the existence of a force he termed **Hahnemannism**.

Hering's criteria, Hering's law, Hering's rule

See: **direction of cure**

heuristic

● Philosophy

Learning from experience. Finding out for oneself.

See also: **empirical**

Etymology: Gk *heurisko* find

hierarchy

● Case taking and analysis, Symptomatology

Pre-arranged sequence of abstract or concrete entities

whose order depends on their lesser or greater effect or importance.

Etymology: Gk *hieros* sacred + *arkhes* ruler

hierarchy of symptoms

● Case taking and analysis, Philosophy, Symptomatology

The arrangement of symptoms in order according to their relative importance in homeopathic case analysis and prescribing; the order of the relative importance of symptoms within the **totality of symptoms**. For example, **strange, rare and peculiar symptoms** are held to be particularly important because of their highly individual character. **Mental** and emotional symptoms usually take precedence over **general symptoms**. **Local** physical symptoms rank lowest in the hierarchy.

Comment:
The concept owes its origin to **Kent** and other homeopaths who, influenced by the philosophy of **Swedenborg**, described a hierarchy in which symptoms of the will and the spirit were of the highest importance, with physical symptoms less important. This particular **doctrine** is popular, but by no means universally applied in contemporary homeopathy.

See also: **evaluation of symptoms, symptom selection**

high dose effect

● Biophysics and biochemistry, Pharmacology and drug action

The biological response to high doses as contrasted with the **low dose effect**. It is exemplified by the **Arndt-Schulz law, biphasic activity** and **hormesis**.

Comment:
It is only of relevance to homeopathy as another example of a type of biphasic biological activity of a

drug. It is in no sense related to the concept of high
and low **potency**.

high potency

See: **potency, high**

histiotropism

See: **tissue affinity**
Etymology: Gk *histos* web + *tropikos* turning

Hippocrates

● Biography, History, Philosophy

Greek physician and philosopher (c. 460–377 BC).
He is known as the 'Father of Medicine' because the
first systematically recorded accounts of the principles
and practice of medicine originated with him and
a number of authors writing in the Hippocratic
tradition. He believed that **health** was a state of
equilibrium, and **illness** a state of disturbed
equilibrium, and focused on the 'dis-ease' rather than
on **disease** as a defined entity. He encouraged close
and frequent observation of the development of the
disease process in the patient, and required attention
to the patient's lifestyle, diet, occupation and
environment. Hippocrates observed that disease could
be eliminated by medicines that caused the same
symptoms.
See also: **Sydenham**

history

● Case taking and analysis

Record or study of past events, as in **patient history**.
See also: **case**
Etymology: Gk *historia* narrative, finding out (*histor*
learned, wise man)

holism

● Philosophy

The principle of regarding organisms and systems

as a whole; as more than the sum of their parts.

See also: **cure, entelechy, healing, health, homeopathic diagnosis**

Etymology: Gk *holos* whole, entire

homeodote

● Pharmacology and drug action, Therapeutics

One homeopathic medicine used as an **antidote** to the effects of another on the basis of the similarity of its **symptom picture** to the symptoms produced by the first medicine.

Etymology: Gk *homoios* like + *doton* given

homeopathic aggravation

See: **therapeutic aggravation**

homeopathic diagnosis

● Case taking and analysis

1 The nature of the **illness** as interpreted in homeopathic practice; a broader interpretation of **diagnosis** than represented by the prevailing pathological **model** in western medicine. It may integrate a number of etiological, personal and clinical factors into a **holistic** perspective of the patient's condition.

2 An **individualised** view of the illness directed towards the choice of an individualised homeopathic medicine; often applied to the choice of homeopathic medicine whose **drug picture** encompasses the whole clinical picture, and expressed in terms of the chosen medicine. In this sense, the concept of **differential diagnosis** may also be applied to the choice between a number of possible homeopathic prescriptions indicated by the **case analysis**.

homeopathic drug

See : **homeopathic medicine**

homeopathic immunotherapy

See: **isopathy**

See also: **immunotherapy**

homeopathic medicinal product

● Pharmacy

A homeopathic medicine in its final form and **potency** ready for administration.

Comment:

1 The wideranging definition given in UK Statutory Instrument SI 1995/308 is as follows: 'Homeopathic medicinal product means a medicinal product (which may contain a number of principles) prepared from products, substances or compositions called homeopathic stocks in accordance with a homeopathic manufacturing procedure described by the European Pharmacopoeia or, in the absence thereof, by any pharmacopoeia used officially in a EU member state.'

homeopathic medicine

● Medical methods

1 The **homeopathic** system of medical practice; its clinical and therapeutic method.

2 The homeopathic prescription. The term preferred in this dictionary, and by the *British Homoeopathic Journal*, for **homeopathic remedy** or homeopathic drug.

homeopathic pathogenetic trial

● Materia medica, Pharmacology and drug action, Research

Experimental procedure for testing substances administered in their natural form, in mother tincture or in potency to healthy volunteers, to elicit effects (**signs**, **symptoms**, changes in behaviour) from which the therapeutic potential or **materia medica** of the substance may be inferred.

Comment:
This term is being increasingly used in place of
proving, an anglicisation of **Hahnemann**'s original
term for the procedure, Prüfung.

Synonyms: **drug proving, experimental
pathogenesis.**

See also: **drug picture, law of similars,
pathogenesis, prover**

homeopathic remedy

● Pharmacology and drug action, Pharmacy,
Therapeutics

The term commonly and colloquially used amongst
homeopaths for the homeopathic medicine because it
implies both the more comprehensive remedial action
which the prescription is expected to achieve and a
more purposive relationship to what is to be remedied
in the patient than the more general term 'medicine'.
The traditional term for the homeopathic prescription
or the homeopathic medicine, the latter being the
term preferred in this dictionary, and by the *British
Homoeopathic Journal.*

Comment:

1 We have to distinguish the pharmaceutical definition
and the medicinal (homeopathic) definition of
homeopathic 'remedies': In the pharmaceutical sense
they are medicines prepared from a variety of **source
materials** according to the principles and procedures
stated in the various official homeopathic
pharmacopeias. This definition does not, however,
depend upon the similarity between the patient's
symptoms and the **drug picture** of the medicine. In
the medicinal sense, therefore, a medicine can be
stated to be truly homeopathic only if the drug
picture corresponds to the presenting **disease
picture** in accordance with the **similia principle.**

2 Another meaning applied to the term, but less
reliable as a definition, is that they are medicines
used according to the principles of Samuel
Hahnemann. Several other ways of using

homeopathy have emerged since Hahnemann's time, however; **drainage therapy** for example. Complex, or **combination remedies** have never been subject to **provings** (although their constituents may have been proven individually), and therefore cannot be administered as the **simillimum. Mother tinctures** are generally considered to be homeopathic, but many have not been proven either and are sometimes described as **herbal medicines**; however the extraction process and vehicles used generally differ so that herbal and homeopathic versions of the same specimen will have different properties.

Synonym: **homeopathic drug**

homeopathicity

● Therapeutics

The state in which the perfect relation or true **similarity** between the **disease picture** and the **drug picture** is said to have been established, usually retrospectively in a **cured** case.

homeopathy

● Medical methods, Philosophy

A therapeutic method using preparations of substances whose effects when administered to healthy subjects correspond to the manifestations of the disorder (symptoms, clinical signs, pathological states) in the individual patient. The method was developed by Samuel **Hahnemann** (1755–1843) and is now practised throughout the world.

Comment:
It is often wrongly supposed that the dilute state of the medicines is the defining characteristic of homeopathy. The defining characteristic is the correspondence described above, known as the **similia principle.** However, the legal definition of homeopathic medicine in France specifies the **potentising** method. See the distinction made between the

pharmaceutical and medicinal definitions of
homeopathic remedy.

See also: **materia medica, proving**

Etymology: Gk *homoios* like + *patheia* suffering

homeopsoric

See: **antipsoric**

homeostasis

● Healing processes, Physiology

1 The state of dynamic equilibrium maintained
within an organism by adjusting its physiological
processes and biochemical mechanisms to changing
circumstances.

2 The process of self-regulation that maintains this
equilibrium.

See also: **autoregulation**

Etymology: Gk *homoios* like + *sta-* stand, *stasis*
standing

homeosycotic

See: **antisycotic**

homeosyphilitic

See: **antisyphylitic**

homoeopathic, homoeopathy

See: **homeopathic, homeopathy** in all entries

homotoxicology

● Medical methods

An interpretation of illness and disease in terms of
the body's inability to cope effectively with the
burden of **toxins** inflicted upon it by diet, life style,
drugs, environment etc., or resulting from
disordered physiological processes. Developed by
Hans Heinrich Reckeweg (1905–1985), it has no
direct connection with homeopathy, but
homeopathic medicines (usually **combination**

remedies) may be used amongst other forms of treatment.

See also: **antihomotoxic therapy**

hormesis

● Biophysics and biochemistry, Pharmacology and drug action

Stimulatory or beneficial effect on an organism of small doses of a toxic substance which in larger doses is inhibitory.

See also: **antitaxic drug action, Arndt-Schulz law, biphasic activity**

Etymology: Gk *hormesis* rapid motion, *horme* impulse

Hughes, Richard

● Biography

English homeopathic physician (1836–1902), and exponent of **low potency** and **pathological prescribing**. He recognised **disease** entities and insisted that homeopathy must take account of the site of action and of pathology. He maintained that **provings** were only valid if conducted with **material doses**, except when **high potency** provings were also supported by **low potency** proving data, and criticised **Hahnemann** for using symptoms derived from the sick. He co-edited the *Cyclopaedia of Drug Pathogenesy* which was published jointly by the **British Homoeopathic Society** and the **American Institute of Homeopathy**. In it all known provings, excluding these carried out by Hahnemann himself, were reviewed in accordance with his strict criteria. His *Manual of Pharmacodynamics* was the leading textbook of **materia medica** in Britain in the late 19th century.

hybrid

See: **mongrel**

hypersensitivity

● Pathology, Physiology

1 An abnormally high degree of bodily sensitivity to a stimulus, resulting in an abnormal or exaggerated response; an exaggerated response of the immune system to the stimulus of a foreign agent.

2 Extreme emotional sensitivity.

See also: **constitution, idiosyncrasy, sensitivity, side-effect**

hypothesis

● Philosophy, Research

1 Statement that predicts or explains a phenomenon, but which is not known to be true.

2 Conjecture offered as a basis for argument or discussion.

3 Proposition offered as the basis for further investigation; which is capable of being tested by experiment.

Comment:
The term has many shades of meaning, depending on the context in which it is used, such as law, logic, philosophy, science. In the context of explaining and validating the principles of homeopathy, the third definition applies.

Etymology: Gk *hupothesis* foundation (*hupo* under + *tithenai* place)

i

iatrogenic

● Disease processes, Therapeutics

Consequence of medical intervention; produced by medical intervention. Hence, iatrogenic illness: illness resulting from medical intervention.

Comment:
The claim that homeopathy does not cause iatrogenic illness, or less politely that 'at least it does no harm', is a **hypothesis** that awaits thorough investigation. Although there is little evidence that homeopathic medicines can cause **adverse drug reactions**, the possibility requires more specific investigation. There are also potential indirect risks associated with homeopathic treatment (see **risk**).

See also: **new symptoms**

Etymology: Gk *iatros* doctor + *genic* produced by

idiosyncrasy

● Constitution, morphology and terrain

1 **Characteristic** that is highly individual and usually rare.
2 In pharmacology, an abnormal and usually uncommon reaction to a drug.

See also: **individuality, adverse drug reaction**

Etymology: Gk *idiosunkrasia* (*idios* own + *sun* together + *krasis* mixture)

illness

● Disease processes

1 Ailment; a state of poor **health.**
2 Disorder of mind or body, not necessarily represented by observable abnormalities of structure or function.

Comment:
In colloquial and in medical usage the terms illness and **disease** are sometimes used interchangeably. The term 'illness', however, has a more general meaning than the term 'disease', encompassing the subjective perception of disorder regardless of any detectable abnormality.
Etymology: ON *illr* bad + OE *ness* state of

immune system

● Physiology

An intricate system of physiological processes which provides the organism with response to and a defence (the immune response) against foreign organisms or substances, and against cells of the organism itself which develop aberrant characteristics.
Etymology: L *immunis* exempt from service (*munis* ready for service)

immunisation

● Physiology, Therapeutics

Protection from or resistance to infectious diseases, conferred by exposure to the infecting organism or its administration in a modified form, or by administration of an inactivated **toxin** (e.g. tetanus).
See also: **immunotherapy, vaccine, vaccinosis**

immunotherapy

● Medical methods

Treatment to enhance the function of the **immune system**. For example, immunisation with a pathogen is 'active immunotherapy'; administering antibodies from another source to counteract the disease in the patient is 'passive immunotherapy'.

Comment:
1 The apparent benefit of homeopathy in many disorders of immunity suggests that one of its pathways of action may be of this nature.
2 'Homeopathic immunotherapy' is used as a synonym for isopathy.

imponderabilia

● Materia medica

Homeopathic medicines prepared from sources which have no material substance, such as electricity, magnetism or X-rays.

Etymology: L *im-* without + *pondus* weight (*ponderare* weigh)

incidental symptom

● Symptomatology

Symptom elicited by enquiry; not included in the presenting problem.

See also: **accessory symptom, complaint, concomitant symptom**

incompatible

See: **inimical**

indication

● Therapeutics
1 That which indicates (points out, shows, suggests or calls for) a particular course of action.
2 A reason for choosing a particular medical intervention, usually a sign, symptom or pathological finding.
3 Less commonly, a pointer to a particular state, condition or diagnosis.

Comment:
1 In homeopathy any sufficiently distinctive feature of the case **history**, though more usually a complex of such features, may provide an indication for the homeopathic prescription.

2 See **alternating symptoms** for an example of a symptom pattern providing indications for a specific homeopathic medicine.

See also: **keynote symptoms, guiding symptoms, individualisation**

Etymology: L *index* forefinger, sign, informer

indisposition

● Disease processes, Therapeutics

Slight ailment or malaise that can be remedied by a change of diet or habit of life, or some similar aspect of behaviour.

individualisation

● Philosophy, Symptomatology, Therapeutics

1 The process of giving individual character to a thing.

2 The art of selecting the homeopathic prescription that corresponds to the particular manifestation of the **illness** in the individual patient rather than on the common characteristics of the **disorder** itself.

See also: **characteristic, constitution, evaluation of symptoms, idiosyncrasy, prescribing strategy, symptom selection**

Etymology: L *in-* un + *dividuus* (*dividere* to divide)

individualised isopathy

See: **autoisopathy**

infinitesimal dose

● Pharmacology and drug action

Dose of medicine whose source material has been diluted beyond **Avogadro's number** and is very unlikely to contain any molecules of the original active ingredient.

See also: **ultrahigh dilution, ultramolecular doses**

information

● Biophysics and biochemistry

Knowledge communicated between people or other

organisms or communication systems or contained in some document or other source. The properties imparted to the homeopathic medicine by the process of **potentisation** may be described hypothetically as a type of information.

See also: **bioenergetics, bioinformation, dynamis, dynamisation, information medicine hypothesis, potency energy**

information medicine hypothesis

● Biophysics and biochemistry

Hypothesis that water and possibly other polar solvents can under certain conditions retain information about other substances with which they have previously been in contact, and which can be imparted to a sensitised biosystem.

See also: **bioinformation, clathrate, cluster, memory of water, solvation structure**

inhalation of medicine

See: **olfaction**

inhibition of potency

See: **destruction of potency**

inimical

● Materia medica, Pharmacology and drug action, Therapeutics

1 Hostile, harmful, unsympathetic.
2 A homeopathic medicine which interferes with the action of another; which has a contrary action to it; but which does not **antidote** it.

Comment:
Homeopathic and conventional medicines are not necessarily inimical when used together.

Synonym: **incompatible** (some countries)
Etymology: LL *inimicalis* (*in-* + *amicus* friend)

initial action

See: **primary drug action**

initial aggravation, initial reaction

See: **therapeutic aggravation**
See also: **primary drug action**

injection of medicine

● Therapeutics

An occasional **route of administration** of homeopathic medicines: either subcutaneous, intramuscular or intravenous. Frequently used in Germany. The method is regarded by some homeopaths as encouraging a better response when the injection site has a neuroanatomical relationship to the affected organ, or is directly adjacent to it, for example around the affected joint.

See also: **dosage form**

integrated medicine

● Medical methods, Therapeutics

The use of different **therapies**, including both **complementary medicine** and **conventional medicine**, and different healthcare agencies and practitioners, in a coordinated and mutually supportive programme of care for the greatest benefit of the individual patient.

See also: **adjuvant therapy**
Synonym: **integrative medicine**

integrative medicine

See: **integrated medicine**

intercurrent remedy

● Therapeutics

One homeopathic medicine used in conjunction with another in a treatment regime, but not at the same time, and usually on the basis of a different set of

indications to the first, or a subset of those indications.

See also: **alternating remedy, major remedy, minor remedy, pluralist homeopathy**

Etymology: L *inter* between + *currere* to run

intermittent diseases

● Disease processes

1 Diseases which recur at definite intervals.
2 Diseases in which one disease state alternates with another from time to time.

See also: **alternating symptoms, periodicity, suppression, syndrome shift, vicariation**

Etymology: L *inter* between + *mittere* to let go

intervention

● Therapeutics

1 An action that comes between; that occurs in the time between two other events, or that modifies the course or result of an event.
2 An act performed with the intention of producing a particular effect. In the context of medicine and health care this includes **treatments**, procedures, regimens or services intended to modify disease processes or physiological or pathological variables, or to change the circumstances which are adversely affecting the patient's **health**.

Etymology: L *inter* between + *venire* to come

intolerance

● Symptomatology

1 Unable or unwilling to bear with or endure something.
2 Adverse reaction to something commonly tolerated by others e.g. foods, medicines (including homeopathic) or circumstances. To be distinguished from **aversion**.

Comment:
Patients often describe intolerance as **allergy**.
Intolerance includes allergy but is a broader concept.

See also: **aggravation, hypersensitivity, idiosyncrasy, sensitivity, tolerance**

Etymology: L *in-* + *tolerare* to endure

isopathic

● Pharmacology and drug action, Therapeutics

Pertaining to **isopathy**.

isopathy

● Pharmacology and drug action, Therapeutics

The use of medicines derived from the causative agent of the disease itself, or from a product of the disease process, to treat the condition. Isopathic medicines include organisms and allergens. For example, *Herpes simplex* **nosode** to treat cold sores, or pollens to treat hayfever. Isopathic medicines do not conform to the principles of homeopathy in that they have not been subjected to **proving**, and are not **individualised**. See **allopathy** for a further account of the difference between isopathy, homeopathy and allopathy.

Comment:

1 The term was probably first used in around 1832 by Wilhelm **Lux**, Professor of Veterinary Science at the University of Leipzig. After initially becoming an enthusiastic homeopath, Lux became convinced that every contagious disease had the means of curing itself and subsequently used isopathic medicines prepared according to homeopathic principles.

2 **Hahnemann** initially expressed interest in the method, suggesting that the **potentised** preparation was changed in the process, and no longer the same as in its original state, and therefore was acting homeopathically, but later he repudiated it.

See also: **autohemic therapy, autoisopathy, autonosode, nosode, sarcode, tautopathy**

Etymology: Gk *isos* equal + *patheia* suffering

itch diathesis

● Disease processes

A pattern of **morbidity** characterised by itching and scabby or scaly skin eruptions, but affecting the whole person. Identified by **Hahnemann** as the primary manifestation of the **psoric miasm**. At the time it was associated with 'scabies', which was then a **diagnosis** that applied to a variety of skin conditions, and not the infestation with *Sarcoptes scabiei* var. *hominis*, with its resulting eruption and itching that it now describes.

j

Jahr, Georg H G

● Biography

German physician (1800–1876), friend and co-worker of **Hahnemann**. Studied homeopathy and became a skilled prescriber before undertaking formal medical training. Became Hahnemann's assistant in the production of *Chronic Diseases*. He was a witness to Hahnemann's death. Maintained that the stronger the most characteristic, and in particular the more **peculiar** the symptoms were, the greater the receptivity of the patient to the homeopathic stimulus, and the higher the most suitable **potency** was likely to be.

Jenichen, Julius Caspar

● Biography, History

Non-medically-qualified homeopath (1787–1845); originally Master of the Horse to the Duke of Gotha, although his enemies pejoratively referred to him as an ostler. He devised a form of very high **potency** in which **dilution** was much reduced and **succussion**, which he regarded as the important component of the process, greatly increased. He gave up to 30 shakes per degree of potency but diluted only after each 25 degrees. He prepared remedies up to the 60 000th. Though denounced by **Hahnemann** at the time, his potencies were later favoured by some homeopathic physicians, including **Hering**, but were again

denounced by others, particularly **Hughes** and
Dudgeon. They enjoyed some popularity until
replaced by the machine-made **millesimal potencies**.

Julian, O A

● Biography

Influential French homeopathic physician (1910–1984)
who wrote on materia medica and therapeutics.

k

Kent, James Tyler

● Biography

American physician (1849–1916). A graduate of an **eclectic** medical school, he was converted to homeopathy after a dramatic cure of his wife in 1878. He was an ardent advocate of **high potencies** and became the leader of that group of prescribers in the USA. Kent's thought has been very influential in 20th century homeopathy in many parts of the world. Many British homeopaths converted to **Kentian** homeopathy in the 1920s. He is best known for his *Repertory,* and for his *Lectures on Materia Medica* and *Lectures on Homoeopathic Philosophy*.

See also: **hierarchy of symptoms, Kentian philosophy**

Kentian

● Philosophy

Kentian philosophy; a follower of the same.

See: **Kentian philosophy**

Kentian philosophy

● Philosophy

Philosophy of homeopathy expounded by **Kent**. Claimed by Kent and his supporters to derive directly from **Hahnemann**, but owes much to **Swedenborg** and to Kent's own moral ideas.

See also: **doctrine**

keynote symptom

● Symptomatology

1 Symptom highly **characteristic** of a particular medicine.

2 Symptom that provides a strong **indication** for the choice of a particular medicine.

Comment:
There is no clear distinction between keynote symptoms and **guiding symptoms**.

See also: **eliminating symptom**

Korsakov, General Simeon Nicolaevich (or von Korsakoff)

● Biography

Probably the first Russian homeopath (died 1853). Although not a doctor, he was given the task of preparing remedies for Tsar Nicholas 1 when he was travelling. He is known principally for his work with high potencies and the development of the Korsakov method of **potentisation** in 1829. See **Korsakov potency**.

Korsakov potency

● Pharmacy

Method of performing each stage in the process of **serial dilution** in which only one container is used throughout the process (**single glass method**), developed by **Korsakov**.

A first **centesimal potency** (known as 1K or 1cK) is prepared by addition of a measured volume of **mother tincture** to an appropriate volume of diluent (1 part in 100) and thorough **succussion** of the resulting solution. Rather than taking one drop of this potency and transferring it to the next vial sequentially, as in a

Hahnemannian potency, the liquid is removed from the vial by suction or inversion, leaving droplets of solution adhering to the wall of the container. New solvent is then added, the vial succussed, usually 100 times, and the process repeated. The first three dilutions are carried out using alcohol of a strength similar to that included in the mother tincture; subsequent dilutions are in distilled water. Only one vial is used for the whole **potentisation** process. In the case of an insoluble substance, the British Homeopathic Pharmacopeia directs that the first three successive Korsakovian **triturations** are prepared in lactose. Subsequent dilutions are prepared in the liquid **diluent** as above. The number of serial dilutions performed in this manner defines the potency.

Comment:
Until the mid-1950s more than half the potencies used in France were prepared in this way, but by 1965 when homeopathic medicine was included in the French Pharmacopeia (8th edn), the Korsakov method, and almost all potencies above 30c, were made illegal. The method is still widely used. The commonest Korsakov potencies (often written with a c preceding the K) are 6K, 12K, 30K, 200K and 1000K (MK).
See also: **millesimal potency**

Künzli, Jost

● Biography

Swiss **Kentian** homeopathic physician (1915–1992). Studied with **Kent** and was influential in the development of homeopathy in his time. Produced *The General Repertory*, based on Kent's repertory, but highlighting symptoms that he had verified from his own practice.

l

lactose

● Pharmacy

Milk sugar; sugar obtained from milk, compounded of galactose and glucose.

Comment:
Finely powdered lactose is used in the manufacture of unmedicated tablets, individual and bulk powders. It is also used as the **diluent** in the **trituration** process.
See also: **dosage form**
Etymology: L *lac* milk

ladder remedies

● Therapeutics

A series of different homeopathic medicines used in sequence in the treatment of complicated **chronic disease**, whose cumulative action is effective where a single medicine cannot effect a **cure**.
See also: **alternating remedies, compatible, complementary remedy, concordances, following remedy, relationship of remedies**

latent period

● Disease processes, Healing processes

1   The interval between the giving of a stimulus and the response to it.

2 The time between the onset of the **disease process** and its clinical manifestations. For example, the incubation period of an infectious illness.

See also: **onset of illness**

Etymology: L *latere* to be hidden

laterality

● Materia medica, Symptomatology

The side of the body affected by the symptom. The concept includes the involvement of diagonally opposite parts in the upper and lower halves of the body, and the movement or alternation of symptoms from side to side. Some homeopathic medicines are associated with a particular laterality, and hence such features may be important in homeopathic prescribing.

Synonym: **sidedness**

Etymology: L *lateralis* (*latus* side)

law of similars

See: **similia principle**

laws of cure

● Case taking and analysis, Healing processes, Therapeutics

Empirical observations of changes in the patient which indicate a favourable response to homeopathic treatment and the progress of the patient towards recovery (the **direction of cure**). The formulation of these observations is attributed to **Hering**, although he did not view them as a set of 'laws'. Nor are they laws in the formal sense of proven laws of physics such as the laws of thermodynamics.

Synonyms: **Hering's criteria, Hering's law, Hering's rule**

See also: **cure, evolution of the case, palliation, reappearance of old symptoms, suppression**

layers of illness

- Disease processes, Healing processes, Symptomatology

  Separate patterns of disorder, superimposed on one another in chronic disease, that become manifest in the course of homeopathic treatment as each successive layer gives way in response to treatment revealing the one 'below'. Each layer consists of a different **symptom picture**, and is likely to require a different homeopathic prescription. The process has been compared to peeling away the layers of an onion. It is entirely different from the concept of the **level of illness**.

  See also: **alternating symptoms, intermittent diseases, metastasis, suppression, syndrome shift**

lay homeopath

- Practitioner

  Homeopathic practitioner who is not legally licensed or qualified.

  Comment:
  Such practice is illegal in all European states except the UK, Eire and Norway, and in all US states. In some countries and states, special officially recognised licensing arrangements exist for **professional homeopaths**.

  See also: **doctor, non-medically-qualified practitioner, physician**
  Etymology: Gk *laikos* (*laos* people)

level of illness

- Disease processes

  The depth to which the individual is adversely affected by the **illness**. The deepest level of illness involves the integrity, creativity and fulfilment of the personality. More superficial levels interfere proportionately less with this capacity for fulfilment. Major and 'vital' organs are similarly involved in deeper levels of illness. **Case analysis**, interpretation of the illness, **prognosis**, and interpretation of the **response to prescription**, all involve an appreciation of the prevailing levels of illness. The concept originated with **Kent**, and is related to the **hierarchy of symptoms**. It is not adopted by of all schools of homeopathy.

See also: **direction of cure, syndrome shift**

life force

● Philosophy

That force, power or energy which animates (breathes life into, enlivens) the material organism. A metaphysical rather than a biological or biophysical concept.

Comment:

1 **Hahnemann** describes this concept in §9–17 of the *Organon*: 'In health, the spirit-like life force (**autocracy**) that enlivens the material organism as **dynamis**, governs without restriction and keeps all parts of the organism in admirable, harmonious, vital operation, as regards both feelings and functions, so that our indwelling, rational spirit can freely avail itself of this living, healthy instrument for the higher purposes of our existence (§9). The diseased life force imparts to the organism the adverse sensations and irregular functions that we call disease (§11). The life force and the material organism are an indivisible whole; they are one and the same, although in thought, we split this unity into two concepts in order to conceptualise it more easily (§15)' (Hahnemann 1996).

2 Similar concepts of life force are found in many cultures throughout history, for example: qi or ch'i (traditional Chinese medicine), prana (India), ka or ga-ilama (Egypt), lung (Tibet), mana (Hawaii), cheim (Judaism), ruh (Islam), akasha (Hinduism), pneuma and apeiron (Greek philosophy), enormon (**Hippocrates**), **vis medicatrix naturae, entelechy** (Aristotle), Archeus (**Paracelsus**), animal magnetism (Mesmer), and others.

Synonyms: **life energy, life principle, vital energy, vital force, vital principle**

See also: **autoregulation, bioenergy, dynamis, vitalism**

Etymology: referred to in the ***Organon*** as 'Lebenskraft' f. G *Leben* life + *kraft* force, power, energy

lift in potency

See: **step**

liquid potency

● Pharmacy

A **potentised** preparation in liquid form, usually a water–alcohol vehicle. May be administered in this form or used to medicate a solid **dosage form**.

LM potency

● Pharmacy

Potencies based on a **dilution** factor of 1/50 000, as compared with 1/10 (**decimal potency**) and 1/100 (**centesimal potency**).

The LM **mother tincture** is prepared from the **C3 trituration** of the source material dissolved in an ethanol and water mixture. From that point, successive potencies are prepared by **serial dilutions** of 1/50 000, with **succussion**.

The potency was introduced by Hahnemann to improve patients' tolerance of repeated doses in chronic disease by increasing the dilution ratio of each potentising step and changing the **potency** of the daily doses. The benefits claimed for this method are that the medicines are less likely to cause **therapeutic aggravation**, and are more deeply acting. The method was not generally known until the publication of the posthumous 6th edition of the ***Organon***, and Hahnemann himself did not give them the name LM. The term is derived from the Latin numerals L (50) and M (1000), although the Latin numeral LM actually means 950. It was for this reason that the term **Q potency** (quinquagintamillesima) was introduced later.

Details of the method for preparing, dispensing and administering the potencies vary, and greater consensus in these matters is desirable. However, the medicine is usually administered in liquid form, and each dose further succussed and diluted before it is taken (**plussing**), thus slightly changing the potency or **dynamisation**.

See also: **Hahnemannian potency, Korsakov potency, millesimal potency, plussing**

Synonym: **Q potency**

local symptom

● Symptomatology

Clinical feature (**symptom** or **sign**) expressing the local manifestation of the illness in relation to a particular organ, system or part of the body. Although **mental symptoms** are always an important component of the **totality of symptoms**, a mental or emotional symptom is a 'local' symptom of a psychological illness.

See also: **general symptom, particular symptom**

local treatment

● Therapeutics
1 Treatment of the **local symptoms**.
2 Treatment with local (topical) applications, or internally, e.g. by injection at the affected site.

See also: **dosage form, injection of medicine, route of administration**

London Homoeopathic Hospital

● History

Established by **Quin** in 1849. Later became the Royal London Homoeopathic Hospital, now the largest public sector homeopathic hospital in Europe.

longilinear constitution

See: **phosphoric constitution**

Loschmidt's number

● Biophysics and biochemistry

The number of elementary particles (atoms in elements or molecules in compounds) in 1 ml of gas at 0°C and 1 atmosphere of pressure. Approximately 2.687 x 10^{19} particles per ml.

Comment:
The Viennese physicist Josef Loschmidt (1821–1895) calculated the constant in 1865. It is similar to **Avogadro's number** and the two are sometimes used synonymously, but Avogadro's number relates to the number of particles in one mole of a substance as opposed to one millilitre.

low dose effect

● Biophysics and biochemistry, Pharmacology and drug action

The biological response to low doses as contrasted with the **high dose effect**. The contrast is exemplified in **biphasic activity**, the **Arndt-Schulz Law** and the phenomenon of **hormesis**.

Comment:
The distinction between high and low doses is related to the toxicity or effective dose of the original material. Thus a high dose of a nontoxic substance such as *Natrum muriaticum* (sodium chloride) would be much larger than that of *Arsenicum album* (arsenous trioxide). It is only of relevance to homeopathy as another example of a type of biphasic biological activity of a drug. It is in no sense related to the concept of high and low **potency**.

See also: **change of phase, dose-dependent reverse effect**

low potency

See: **potency, low**

lues

See: **syphilitic miasm**

Etymology: L *lues* pestilence, plague

luetic miasm

See: **syphilitic miasm**

Lux, Johann Wilhelm

● Biography

German pioneer of **veterinary homeopathy** (1776–1849). In 1833 he published *Isopathik der Contagion* in which he advocated **isopathy**, suggesting that every disease carried the key to its own cure.

m

M potency

See: **millesimal potency**

macerate

- Pharmacy
1 To soften by soaking.
2 The process by which a plant is caused to disintegrate by soaking in an appropriate solvent vehicle with or without the application of heat.

Comment:
Examples of suitable vehicles are water, water–ethanol, glycerol. The solid residue is removed by filtration, and the active principles remain in solution to provide the **stock** or **mother tincture** for a homeopathic medicine. A water–ethanol vehicle is commonly used for preparing homeopathic medicines

Etymology: L *macerare* soak, soften, weaken

maintaining cause

See: **obstacle to cure**

major remedy

- Materia medica, Therapeutics
1 A homeopathic medicine with deep acting or wide

ranging effects, but not necessarily the full spectrum of activity of a **polychrest**.

2 A homeopathic medicine used as the main prescription when another **minor remedy** is used as an **intercurrent remedy**.

See also: **frequently used remedy**

malaria

● Disease processes, History

A disease caused by the infestation of red blood cells by the protozoa of the genus *Plasmodium*. Usually transmitted between humans by the bite of an infected female *Anopheles* mosquito. Previously attributed to the unhealthy air, or noxious emanation (literally **miasm**) arising from marshy land. Still **endemic** in certain parts of the world. The condition whose treatment with **cinchona bark** stimulated **Hahnemann**'s interest in the possibility of curing like with like.

Synonym: **marsh fever**

Etymology: It *mala* bad + *aria* air

marsh fever

See: **malaria**

materia medica

● Main category, Therapeutics

1 Systematic documentation of the knowledge of medicines; a textbook containing such.

2 The scientific study of the sources, preparation, uses and administration of medicines.

3 In homeopathy, the description of the nature and therapeutic repertoire of homeopathic medicines; of the pathology, the symptoms and signs and their modifying factors (**modalities**), and the general characteristics of the patient associated with them, derived from their **toxicology**, **homeopathic**

pathogenetic trials (**provings**) and clinical experience of their use.

4   The intrinsic characteristics of the **source material**.

See also: **drug picture, guiding symptoms, homeopathic pathogenetic trial, key note symptoms, pharmacognosy, pharmacology, repertory**

Materia Medica Pura

● Materia Medica

Hahnemann's principal treatise on homeopathic **materia medica** (1811–1821, 2nd edn 1825–1833). Symptoms are presented as described by the volunteer (**prover**), although some are derived from **toxicology**.

See also: **homeopathic pathogenetic trial, materia medica, proving**

Etymology: L *materia* subject of discourse

material dose

● Pharmacy, Therapeutics

A dose which contains a measurable amount of the source material.

Synonym: **ponderal dose, substantial dose**

See also: **Avogadro's number, concentration, dilution, infinitesimal dose, ultrahigh dilution, ultramolecular dilution**

Etymology: L *materia* timber, substance

mechanistic

● Philosophy

The belief that all natural phenomena, including life, **illness** and **healing** processes, can be explained mechanically; that is, in terms of physics and chemistry.

Etymology: Gk *mekhanikos* (*mekhos* contrivance)

medical homeopath

● Practitioner

Officially licensed doctor practising homeopathy.

See also: **lay homeopath, non-medically-qualified homeopath, professional homeopath**

medical model

See: **biomedical model**

medicating potency

● Pharmacy

The **liquid potency** used to medicate solid and liquid **dosage forms**.

memory of water

● Biophysics and biochemistry

The hypothetical property of water and water–ethanol mixtures to be able to carry and transmit **information**; a biologically active message or imprint imposed upon them during the process of **potentisation**.

Comment:
The term was coined to describe the properties revealed in controversial experiments by the French immunologist, Jacques Benveniste, on the activity of homeopathic **potencies**. If this hypothesis is valid, however, it could be used to justify the argument that the water–ethanol vehicle actually becomes the active principle, rather than the adjuvant.
See also: **clathrate, cluster, information medicine hypothesis, solvation structures**

mental symptom

● Case taking and analysis, Symptomatology

Characteristic of the mental state of the patient when he or she is ill, irrespective of whether the presenting features of the **illness** involve the mind or emotions; mental and emotional symptoms that characterise a specific **clinical picture** (e.g. fear of death during a panic attack), rather than aspects of the individual's usual personality or **constitution** (e.g. a habitual tendency to worry). The concept of mental symptoms in homeopathy embraces consciousness, intellect, thinking and reasoning, and **emotion**, and any disorder of these faculties.

Synonym: **mind symptom**

See also: **hierarchy of symptoms, general symptom, local symptom**

metastasis

● Disease processes

The transfer or spread of a **disease process** or its manifestations, or of the causative agent (e.g. an organism) from one organ or part of the body to another. The concept is most commonly associated with the spread of cancer cells through the body from the original site.

Comment:

In **conventional medicine**, metastasis usually represents the progression of the disease process. In homeopathic thinking, metastases can be caused by the self-regulating, protective action of the **life force** shifting the disease process to less vital organs, whereas metastasis in the more destructive sense may be attributed to **allopathic** treatment, which may cause **suppression** of a disease process, as well as the progression of the disease itself.

See also: **direction of cure, level of illness, suppression, syndrome shift, vicariation**

Etymology: Gk *methistemi* change

miasm

● Disease processes, Philosophy, Therapeutics

1 Infectious or noxious vapour or atmosphere.
2 Pathogenic influence of a particular **disease process** upon an organism, responsible for a wide but distinctive range of **morbidity** not necessarily characteristic of the pathology of the original disease.
3 **Trait** within a society, family or individual making them susceptible to a particular pattern of morbidity;

an inherited or acquired **disposition** to be ill in a certain way.

Comment:

1 A complex concept which has evolved throughout the history of homeopathy. Originally attributed by **Hahnemann** to the acquired or inherited effects of three diseases, 'itch' (**psora**), gonorrhea (**sycosis**) and **syphilis** (or lues), they have become associated in recent times with more generic categories of disorder. These are deficiency or underreaction (psora), excess or overreaction (sycosis) and breakdown or disorganisation (syphilis). Interpretation of the hereditary, acquired and environmental components of the miasmatic state vary. Later additions to these classes of miasm are the **tubercular diathesis** and cancerinic miasm.

2 The concept of miasm has always been controversial, even more so in the context of modern scientific understanding of disease processes. It is not accepted by all homeopaths, many of whom practise without reference to it. Nevertheless, it is influential in **classical homeopathy**, and an aspect of the **model** of health and illness that homeopathy presents which merits investigation.

See also: **constitution, diathesis, predisposition, psoric miasm, sycotic miasm, syphilitic miasm, terrain**

Etymology: Gk *miasma* defilement, pollution

miasmatic trait

● Disease processes

A **characteristic** or **trait** in the health history, personality, **constitution** or family background of an individual that is associated with a particular **miasm**.

milk sugar

See: **lactose**

Miller, R Gibson

● Biography

Scottish physician (1862–1919) who studied with **Kent** in America, and formulated a comprehensive table of the **relationship of remedies**.

millesimal potency

● Pharmacy

Theoretically, a **dilution** in the proportion of 1 part in 1000; the addition of 1 part of the stock or of the previous **potency** in a sequence to 999 parts of **diluent**. The number of **steps** or **serial dilutions** performed in this manner, with **succussion**, defines the millesimal potency. They are usually prepared by the **Korsakov** method, though starting from a low **centesimal potency** such as the **C3 trituration**.

Comment:

1 There is disagreement as to whether this is a legitimate **potency scale**, and to what extent these potencies are available, manufactured or used.

2 The **Korsakov** method, using a **single glass** container for each **step** in the process to dilute the residue of the previous potency remaining on the walls of the container when it has been emptied, has two consequences. One is that the dilution ratio of 1/1000 may not be precise, although it can be made reasonably accurate by adjusting the geometry of the vessel. The other is that molecules of the original **source material** may persist due to adhesion to the walls of the container.

See also: **centesimal potency, decimal potency, Hahnemannian potency, Korsakov potency, LM potency, potency scale**

Etymology: L *mille* thousand

mind symptom

See: **mental symptom**

minimum dose

● Therapeutics

The smallest dose of a homeopathic medicine that will produce the desired therapeutic effect.

Etymology: L *minimus* smallest, least

minimum symptoms of maximum value

● Symptomatology, Therapeutics

The few symptoms of exceptional value which most clearly allow **individualisation** of the **case**; which express the **centre of the case**.

Etymology: L *minimus* smallest, least

minor remedy

● Materia medica, Therapeutics

1　A homeopathic medicine whose **drug picture** is limited; a medicine with relatively few known characteristics and **indications**.

2　A medicine that has not been subjected to extensive **proving**, and whose full therapeutic potential is not yet known.

3　A medicine used as an **intercurrent remedy** in a regime with a **major remedy**, corresponding to the local symptoms or to a circumscribed pattern of symptoms.

Synonym: **small remedy**

See also: **frequently used remedy, major remedy, polychrest, status of medicines**

Etymology: L *minuere* lessen

modality

● Materia medica, Symptomatology, Therapeutics

1　The mode, form or manner of a procedure (as in **therapeutic modality**).

2　In homeopathy, a factor which modifies the behaviour, level, degree of intensity or severity of a clinical state (symptom, sign, pathology or disorder). This may be: another clinical condition, a physiological function, an emotional state, an activity, the behaviour of the patient, food and drink, time of day, any experience or circumstance, including **environmental factors**, to which the patient is exposed, or commonplace **palliative** measures or reactions such as rubbing or scratching. It does not include the effect of specific therapeutic interventions. Of great importance in homeopathy in describing a **complete symptom**.

See also: **aggravation, amelioration, contradictory modality, environmental factors, temperature modality, time modality, weather modality**

Etymology: L *modalitas* f. *modalis* (*modus* measure)

model

● Medical methods, Philosophy

Conceptual framework used to represent a dynamic system. Hence **biomedical model**, the conceptual framework used to represent the phenomenon of illness and healing in **conventional medicine**.

Etymology: L *modus* measure

mongrels

● History

Hahnemann's pejorative epithet ('gentlemen of the new mongrel sect') for physicians of his day who called themselves homeopaths, but who took no trouble to select medicines on truly homeopathic principles and usually resorted to **allopathic** treatments as well. Also known as **half homeopaths**.

morbidity

● Disease processes
1 A state of **disease**.
2 The incidence of disease in a population, or in particular circumstances (e.g. following a surgical procedure).

Etymology: L *morbus* disease

morbific

● Disease processes

Pertaining to an agent capable of inducing disease; pathogenic.

Etymology: L *morbus* disease

morphology

● Constitution, morphology and terrain

1 The study and classification of the form of things.
2 In medicine, the study and classification of body form.
3 The basis of one view of **typology** or **constitution** in homeopathy.

See also: **carbonic constitution, fluoric constitution, Grauvogl, Nebel, phosphoric constitution, sulphuric constitution**

Etymology: Gk *morphe* form

mother tincture

● Pharmacy

Liquid preparations resulting from the extraction of suitable **source material** in water–ethanol mixtures, which form the starting point for the production of most homeopathic medicines. Comminution (breaking into fragments), followed by standard **maceration** and squeezing techniques are used on fresh plants and succulents, while dried specimens are subjected mainly to percolation with alcohol on a column. Less commonly the term may be applied to material of a mineral nature (as a starting point for other dilutions) or animal source material.

Comment:
In later life, around 1835, Hahnemann is reported to have stopped preparing potencies from mother tinctures of soluble source material, preferring to process crude plant drugs, **expressed juices** and **fresh plants** by **trituration** with **lactose**.

See also: **herbal medicine, tincture**

multiflask method

See: **multiglass method**

multiglass method

● Pharmacy

Method of producing **serial dilutions** in separate clean glass vials originally used by **Hahnemann**.

Synonym: **multiflask method**

See also: **Hahnemannian potency, Korsakov potency, single glass method**

Mure, Benoit

● Biography

Intrepid French promulagator of homeopathy (1809–1858). Introduced it to Brazil and Egypt. Recommended the use of **low potencies** for acute conditions, and **high potencies** for chronic conditions.

n

Nash, E B

● Biography

American physician (1838–1914); exponent of
keynotes which he described in his *Leaders in
Homoeopathic Therapeutics* (1898).

natural history of disease

● Disease processes

The familiar course of a disease if it is not altered by
medical intervention.

natural medicine

● Medical methods

1   Treatment that depends upon stimulating the
organism's natural abilities for **autoregulation**.
2   Treatment that uses naturally occurring therapeutic
agents such as heat and light, or herbs.

Comment:
The term is rather vague, and sometimes used
synonymously with **complementary medicine** and
alternative medicine, but although a particular
therapeutic method may belong to all three
categories, the distinctive meanings need to be borne
in mind.

naturopathy

● Medical methods

Treatment which uses naturally occurring forces or materials such as light, heat, electricity or diet, or physical methods such as massage to mobilise and reinforce the bodies own self-regulating and self-healing mechanisms and resources.

See also: **autoregulation, autoregulatory therapy**

Nebel, Antoine

● Biography

Leading French homeopath (1870–1954). Noted for his interest in **high potencies** and **typology**, and also a proponent of **drainage** therapy. Developed a description of three constitutional types based on characteristics of physique, the **carbonic**, **fluoric**, and **phosphoric** constitutions, which superseded the earlier classification of **Grauvogl**.

See also: **constitution, morphology, typology**

Neckar, George

● Biography

See: **Quin**

neuropeptide

● Physiology

Peptides involved in the function of the central nervous system. Peptides are compounds of amino-acid residues linked by amide bonds.

Comment:
It is postulated that neuropeptides may mediate the effect of the homeopathic stimulus in some cases.

never well since

● Case taking and analysis, Disease processes, Therapeutics

A statement expressing the relationship between specific events or experiences in the patient's life and the onset of **illness**, possibly but not necessarily the **presenting problem** itself. An **etiological factor** of this kind may be important in choosing the homeopathic prescription or planning the **prescribing strategy**.

See also: **ailments from, causal, causality, causation, precipitating factor**

new symptoms

● Case taking and analysis, Disease processes, Therapeutics

Symptoms never before experienced by the patient. They may be the product of the existing **disease process**, or of some new disease process or intercurrent event, or of the **intervention**, including the response to a homeopathic prescription which is not the true **simillimum** or has produced **proving symptoms**. They must be distinguished from the **reappearance of old symptoms** which has quite different significance.

See also: **iatrogenic, similar**

nocebo effect

● Disease processes, Therapeutics

The adverse effects of **placebos**; the phenomenon in which an inert substance elicits adverse effects in the subject to whom it is administered, as opposed to the beneficial effect of placebo. Unlike placebo, however, which may be administered with deliberate beneficial intent, the nocebo effect is not intended.

Comment:
It has been suggested that patients may experience recurrence of symptoms which have resolved, as a direct result of not receiving the further prescription which they had expected, and that this should be regarded as a nocebo effect.

See also: **non-specific effects**
Etymology: L *nocebo* I will harm

non-medically-qualified practitioner

● Practitioner

Practitioner of some form of therapy, usually an **alternative** or **complementary therapy** who does not hold a statutory medical qualification.

See also: **doctor, lay homeopath, physician, professional homeopath**

non-specific effects

● Healing processes, Research, Therapeutics

The influence of factors other than the specific therapeutic agent or technique upon the outcome of **treatment** or of the **therapeutic encounter**.

See also: **nocebo, placebo**

normolinear constitution

See: **sulphuric constitution**

nosode

● Materia medica, Pharmacy, Therapeutics

Homeopathic medicine derived from pathological material. May be of human, animal or plant origin, including microorganisms, diseased tissue, or the products of disease processes, such as discharges and effusions.

See also: **autoisopathy, autohemic therapy, autonosode, bowel nosode, isopathy**

Etymology: Gk *nosos* disease + *eides* like

nosography

See: **pathography**

nosology

● Disease processes

The systematic classification of diseases; the science of classification of diseases.

Etymology: Gk *nosos* disease + *-logia* subject of study (*logos* account, discourse)

null hypothesis

● Research

In medical research, an experimental hypothesis that different treatments or procedures will have equivalent outcomes, or that the populations concerned do not differ from each other; the proposition that the results of an experiment will not differ from those that might be expected by chance alone. A proposition used to test a **hypothesis**; if rejected, it increases confidence in the hypothesis.

objective

- Symptomatology
1 Pertaining to observable or measurable facts; perception of things external to the mind by use of the senses.
2 Of **symptoms** and **signs**, observed by another and not perceived by the patient alone.

Etymology: L *objectum* thing presented to the mind

obstacle to cure

- Case taking and analysis, Disease processes, Healing processes, Therapeutics

Factor in the nature of the disease process, or in the nature and personality of the individual, or in his or her circumstances, relationships, habits or lifestyle that prevents a response to a well-indicated homeopathic medicine.

Synonym: **maintaining cause**
Etymology: L *ob-* against + *stare* stand

occasion

- Case taking and analysis, Disease processes
1 The time of a particular occurrence.
2 The reason, justification or need for an occurrence.

3 A circumstance that brings about a certain occurrence, usually as an incidental rather than direct cause.

4 In homeopathic thinking, the circumstances contributing to or surrounding the onset of an illness rather than its direct cause or **precipitating factor**.

See also: **biopathography, environmental factors, etiology, onset, never well since, pathogenesis, precipitating factor**

Etymology: L *occasio* juncture

old school

● History, Philosophy

Hahnemann's name for practitioners of the prevailing medical orthodoxy of his day (**allopathy**), which he regarded with contempt for its destructive effects, particularly the **suppression** of the manifestation's of disease which left the fundamental disorder to grow stronger or produce new ailments.

old symptoms

See: **reappearance of old symptoms**

olfaction, olfactory route

● Therapeutics

Inhalation through the nose (smelling or olfaction) is an occasional **route of administration** in which the vapour from homeopathic medicines in liquid (sometimes nebulised) or **powder** form (sometimes as **globuli**) is inhaled through the nose. The method was introduced in 1827 and utilised by **Hahnemann** until his death, but subsequently fell out of favour.

Synonym: **inhalation of medicine**

See also: **route of administration, dosage form**

one-sided case, one-sided disease, one-sided illness

● Disease processes, Symptomatology

1 **Illness** with restricted **symptomatology**; a **clinical**

picture restricted to one organ or body system or dominated by one or two local symptoms, obscuring any others.

2   A case which lacks sufficient symptoms on which to base a reliable prescription.

Synonym: **defective case, paucity of symptoms**

onset of illness

● Disease processes

The nature and circumstances surrounding the onset of an **illness** or **disease**: the pattern of symptoms prevailing at the onset; the rate of onset; the circumstances or life events related to it.

Comment:
In homeopathy, the circumstances and characteristics of the onset of the illness may be of particular significance in understanding its nature and in formulating the treatment strategy.

See also: **biopathography, etiological factor, causality, occasion, fundamental cause, pathogenesis, precipitating factor**

ontology

● Disease processes, Philosophy

A branch of metaphysics that deals with the nature of being; human nature and the nature of things. It relates to our perception of normality and disease, individual identity and values. The ontological model of diseases as discrete entities (real things) emerged strongly in the 16th century, and has antecedents in classical times. Ontology is gaining a place as a branch of contemporary medicine.

Etymology: Gk *ontos* being + *logos* account, discourse

organ affinity

● Materia medica, Pharmacology and drug action, Therapeutics

Specific relationship between a medicine and an organ; tendency of a medicine to act on a specific organ. For example, *Chelidonium* is said to have an organ affinity with the biliary tract.

Synonym: **organotropism**

See also: **affinity, disease affinity, drainage, tissue affinity**

Etymology: L *affinitas* bordering on

Organon

● History, Philosophy

1 In its original Greek and Latin sense, an 'organ'; a morphic unit; any structural united collection of cells that is normally capable of coherently exercising a specific life-furthering function for the benefit of the greater whole – the individual body (Gaier 1991 EDH).

2 An instrument of thought; a system of reasoning or logic; a set of principles for use in scientific or philosophical investigation. Aristotle (384–322 BC) and Francis Bacon (1561–1626) entitled their respective writings on logic and scientific method the *Organon* and *Novum Organum* (*new Organon*).

3 Original statement of the basic paradigm and principles of homeopathic medicine, developed by Samuel **Hahnemann** through a series of six editions from 1810 to 1842.

Comment:

1 The first edition of Hahnemann's *Organon* was entitled *Organon der rationellen Heilkunde* (*Organon of Rational Medicine*). The second and subsequent editions were entitled *Organon der Heilkunst* (*Organon of the Healing (or Medical) Art*).

2 The sixth and final edition, containing important revisions, was completed by Hahnemann in 1842, but was not published until 1921 (by **Haehl**; see **Melanie Hahnemann**); **Boericke** translated the revisions into English, and collated them with **Dudgeon**'s 1849 translation of the fifth edition; this was published in 1922.

Etymology: Gk *organon* instrument, tool (instrument of thought or reason)

organopathy

See: **organotherapy**

organotherapy, organ therapy

● Medical methods

1 In conventional usage, the treatment of disease by preparations made from animal organs; particularly endocrine glands. This practice is now largely superseded by the use of synthetic preparations instead of glandular extracts.

2 Its connection with homeopathy is in the treatment of disorder of a particular organ with **potentised** extract of the same healthy organ (technically a **sarcode**). This is not based on **homeopathic** principles, but on the proposition that all **disease** is local and that medicines must affect the same organ as the disease. This contrasted with Hahnemann's **holistic** belief that disease is a general affliction, and was developed by pupils and successors of Hahnemann who found his **doctrine** unacceptable. The concept itself predates **Hahnemann**. The terms 'organopathy' and 'organ therapy' describe the same therapeutic method.

See also: **organ affinity, Rademacher**

organotropism

See: **organ affinity**

orthodox

● Philosophy

Holding the right opinion.

Comment:

1 Often used as synonymous with 'conventional', as in '**conventional medicine**', but the two are not truly equivalent.

2 'Orthodoxy' is so often claimed by separate elements of what is really a wider heterodoxy that it may be better to regard it as a concept that represents a way

of thinking based on discipline and integrity rather than a specific set of ideas.

See also: **conventional medicine, hypothesis, medical model**

Etymology: Gk *orthos* straight, correct, true + *doxa* opinion

oversensitive patient

See: **sensitive type**

p

palliative

● Therapeutics

Treatment that alleviates symptoms without changing
the underlying condition.

Comment:
1 In homeopathy, treatment that has a palliative effect
   is not necessarily regarded as beneficial to the
   patient, and as potentially deleterious if it involves
   suppression of the manifestations of the **disease**;
   palliation of the presenting **complaint** is undesirable if
   accompanied by the appearance or increase of other
   more important symptoms. However, palliative
   homeopathic treatment of incurable diseases such as
   cancer is widely practised.
2 The term 'palliative' is used by **Hahnemann** as
   synonymous with **antipathic**.

See also: **direction of cure**

Etymology: LL *palliare* to cloak

Paracelsus

● Biography

Assumed name of Theophrastus Phillipus Aureolus
Bombastus von Hohenheim, Swiss physician
(1493–1542). Only partially trained in the medical
orthodoxy of his day, he evolved his own idiosyncratic

philosophy of medicine, which incorporated a number of alchemical, mystical and esoteric influences. He had a huge contempt for academia and the medical establishment, and repudiated **Hippocrates** and the **Galenic** concepts of qualities, elements and humours, developing instead a new natural philosophy based on the alchemical 'qualities' of 'salt', 'sulphur' and 'mercury'. Although his theories took medicine one step closer to modern concepts of **ontology** and **pathology**, he nevertheless regarded disease as essentially spiritual. He was an exponent of the **doctrine of signatures**, mistakenly regarded as a forerunner of the **similia principle**. His influence on medicine was by no means only philosophical, however. He was a founder of industrial medicine, and studied the diseases of miners in detail. He introduced the Chinese and Arab practice of using metals and minerals in the treatment of disease to Europe, where herbal medicine had been the norm.

paradoxical symptom

● Symptomatology

A symptom whose behaviour contradicts expectation. For example, a sore throat that is relieved by swallowing solid food.

Etymology: Gk *para-* beyond + *doxa* opinion

paraphrase

● Case taking

Expressing what has been said in other words in order to clarify its accuracy or meaning.

Comment:

An important method of eliciting the meaning of a patient's account of the problem, but of less value than clear spontaneous statements in the **evaluation of symptoms**.

Etymology: Gk *paraphrasis* (*para* beside + *phrazo* tell)

particular symptom

● Symptomatology

Symptom relating to a part of the body.

See also: **local symptom, complaint**

Etymology: L *pars, partis* part

Paschero, Thomas Pablo

● Biography

Argentine radical **unicist** (1904–1986). Developed a contemporary interpretation of the theory of **miasms** with particular emphasis on the influence of environmental rather than inherited factors, and in which original sin is related to the **psoric miasm**.

Paterson, John

● Biography

Scottish physician and bacteriologist (1890–1954), who with his wife Elizabeth continued the work on the **bowel nosodes**, begun by Edward **Bach**.

See also: **Bach flower remedies**

pathogenesis

● Disease processes, Materia medica

1 The pathological, physiological, or biochemical processes resulting in the development of a disease; the progress of an illness through its various stages as it becomes established; 'the march of events' in the development of the disease (**Sydenham**).

2 The progress of an illness from its acute to its chronic manifestation, or from its superficial to its more deep-seated manifestation.

3 The pathological effects of a substance resulting from its natural toxicity or produced in the course of a **homeopathic pathogenetic trial** or **proving**.

Etymology: Gk *pathos* suffering + *genesis* birth

pathogenetic trial

See: **homeopathic pathogenetic trial**

pathognomonic

● Disease processes, Symptomatology

The identifying **characteristics** or indicators of a **disease**; the typical **symptoms**, findings (clinical or laboratory observations), or pattern of abnormalities specific and exclusive to a given disease.

Comment:
Whereas the pathognomonic features of a disease are the most helpful in conventional **diagnosis**, they are usually the least helpful in selecting a homeopathic prescription because they are the least characteristic of the individual expression of the **disease process** in the individual patient.

Etymology: Gk *pathos* suffering + *gnomo* mark, sign, indicator

pathography

● Disease processes

The systematic and detailed description of diseases.

Synonym: **nosography**

Etymology: Gk *pathos* suffering + *-graphos* writing, describing

pathological prescribing

● Therapeutics

Homeopathic prescribing based on pathological indications; the choice of the homeopathic medicine based exclusively on the correspondence of the pathology described in its **materia medica** with the pathology found in the patient, without reference to symptom similarity or other characteristics. An example is the use of *Phosphorus* in the treatment of hepatitis. This contrasts with **Kentian** and other approaches which place great emphasis on **mental symptoms** and **constitution**.

See also: **disease affinity, pathogenesis, pathotropism, specific**

pathology

● Disease processes

1 The systematic study of **disease processes**, from the molecular, genetic and cellular level to the gross, visible morphological changes.

2 The medical science and speciality concerned with all aspects of disease processes, their essential nature, causes, and development.

Etymology: Gk *pathos* suffering + *-logia* subject of study (*logos* account, discourse)

pathotropism

See: **disease affinity**

patient history

● Case taking and analysis

A systematic record of the **illness**, its **evolution** and all attendant and relevant facts and circumstances, provided by the patient or from other sources.

See also: **anamnesis, case taking, catamnesis**

pattern recognition

● Case taking and analysis, Symptomatology

Recognising recurring patterns in events, in behaviour and in the nature of things, including patterns of **symptoms** and **signs** and patient **characteristics**.

Comment:
Part of clinical method in all medicine. Allows the hypothesis that other confirmatory symptoms will be found, which can be tested by further enquiry. An important art or skill in homeopathic **case analysis** for selecting the prescription.

paucity of symptoms

See: **one-sided case**

peculiar

● Symptomatology
1 Exclusively characteristic of; belonging exclusively to.
2 Strange, unusual.
   See: **strange, rare and peculiar symptom**
   Etymology: L *peculiaris* not held in common f. *peculium*
   property (*pecu* herd)

periodicity

● Symptomatology
1 The recurrence of an event at regular intervals.
2 The interval between separate but regular occurrences
   of an event or phenomenon, including episodes of an
   illness or its symptoms.
3 A characteristic feature of the behaviour of symptoms
   in the **materia medica** of some medicines.
   Etymology: Gk *periodos* circuit, recurrence, course

pharmaceutics

   See: **pharmacy**

pharmacodynamics

● Pharmacology and drug action, Therapeutics
1 The study of the behaviour of drugs in living
   organisms; the action of the drug on the body.
2 The uptake, behaviour and interactions of a drug at
   the active site. The presence and concentration of a
   drug at a site in the body is determined by its
   pharmacokinetics.
   Comment:
   The question whether the actions and effects of
   homeopathic medicines are pharmacodynamic is still a
   matter of debate and definition, which may be resolved
   by further research. *The term was used by Hughes in the
   title of his **Manual of Pharmacodynamics**.*
   Etymology: Gk *pharmakon* drug + *dynamis* power

pharmacognosy

● Pharmacology and drug action

The study of crude drugs derived from naturally occurring sources, particularly plants.

Etymology: Gk *pharmakon* drug + *gnosis* knowledge

pharmacokinetics

● Pharmacology and drug action, Therapeutics

The study of the metabolism and action of drugs in the body, as determined by their absorption, distribution and elimination over time; the action of the body on the drug.

See also: **pharmacodynamics**

Etymology: Gk *pharmakon* drug + *kinesis* movement

pharmacology

● Pharmacology and drug action

The science of drugs, their origin, isolation, chemistry, preparation, uses and effects. Embraces aspects of pharmacokinetics and pharmacodynamics, therapeutics and toxicology.

Etymology: Gk *pharmakon* drug + *-logia* subject of study *(logos* account, discourse)

pharmaconomy

See: **posology**

pharmacopeia

● Pharmacology and drug action, Pharmacy

A formal document consisting of monographs describing the composition, properties, manufacture and quality control of drugs. The French and German homeopathic pharmacopeias form part of their official national pharmacopeia. A European homeopathic pharmacopeia is currently in preparation (1999).

Etymology: Gk *pharmakon* drug + *-poios* -making, -maker

pharmacy

● Pharmacy

1   The practice of preparing, formulating and dispensing medicines.
2   The place where medicines are compounded and dispensed.

Synonym: **pharmaceutics**

Etymology: Gk *pharmakeus* druggist, *pharmakeia* practice of druggist

phenomenology

● Philosophy

1   The study, description and classification of phenomena without regard to explanation or interpretation, or to the subjective or objective nature of the experience.
2   The study of all the manifestations of an occurrence rather than of one circumscribed aspect of it or one particular view.

Comment:
Much of homeopathy's approach to **illness** is phenomenological. This is part of its **holistic** perspective. Both characteristics are opposed to the **mechanistic** or **reductionist** tendency inherent in the prevailing **biomedical model**.

Etymology: phainomenon f. phainomai appear, phaino show

philosophy

● Philosophy

1   The search for wisdom and knowledge; especially of ultimate reality and the underlying principles of existence.
2   A system of principles for understanding the nature of things.
3   In homeopathy, the whole theoretical approach to its principles and practice, including both metaphysical concepts and practical aspects of case management.

Comment:
During its history homeopathy has been influenced, sometimes without acknowledgement, by various philosophical systems. These include the influence of **Swedenborg** in 19th-century US homeopathy, and the influence of Freudian and Jungian thought and that of St Thomas Aquinas in the Latin American radical **unicist** school.

Etymology: Gk phileo to love + sophia wisdom

phosphoric constitution

● Constitution, Morphology and terrain

The association described by **Nebel** of tall, lean, supple people with the characteristics of the homeopathic medicine *Calcarea phosphorica*.

Synonym: **longilinear constitution**

See also: **constitution, carbonic constitution, fluoric constitution, morphology, sulphuric constitution, typology**

physician

● Practitioner

One statutorily qualified in the science and art of medicine.

Etymology: Gk one skilled in matters of phusike of nature

picture

● Case taking and analysis, Philosophy, Symptomatology

A metaphor expressing the complete view of a subject that is built up in the study both of an individual patient and of the **materia medica** of a homeopathic medicine.

Comment:
The concept reflects the **phenomenology** and **holism** inherent in the homeopathic approach.

See also: **clinical picture, symptom picture, disease picture, drug picture**

pill, pillule

See: **dosage form**

placebo

● Drug action, Pharmacology, Therapeutics

1 A substance with no active biological properties, knowingly or unknowingly used to exert a beneficial therapeutic effect, or given to satisfy a patient's expectations of treatment.

2 An inactive agent used for comparison with the substance or method to be tested in a controlled trial, and indistinguishable from it.

See also: **nocebo, non-specific effects**

Etymology: L *placebo* I will please

pluralist homeopathy

● Philosophy, Therapeutics

School or **philosophy** of homeopathic therapeutics in which more than one homeopathic medicine representing different aspects of the **illness** are given in a single prescription. The adjective 'pluralist' may describe the practitioner or the method.

Comment:
Although the different medicines are prescribed together the instructions usually require that they are actually taken at different times, as distinct from complex or combination homeopathy which uses fixed mixtures in a single dosage form.

See also: **complex homeopathy, combination remedies, polypharmacy, unicist homeopathy**

Etymology: L *pluralis* (*plus, pluris* more)

plussing

● Pharmacology and drug action, Pharmacy, Therapeutics

The practice of further diluting and succussing homeopathic medicines, or simply resuccussing, before each dose or at intervals during regular **repetition of**

the dose. Plussing is claimed both to reduce **aggravations** and to increase the **potency** of the medicine. It is particularly used with **LM potencies**.

See also: **ascending potencies, dynamisation, potency complex, potentisation, succussion**

Etymology: L *plus* more

polychrest

● Materia medica, Therapeutics

Homeopathic medicine of many uses; whose **drug picture** shows a very wide spectrum of activity in both acute and chronic illness, affecting all or nearly all the tissues of the body and showing a great variety of **symptomatology**, and therefore has a broad range of clinical application. Also used as **constitutional medicines**.

Comment:
1 The term was taken from Greek by Hahnemann and first used by him in an 1817 article on *Nux vomica*.
2 There is debate as to what exactly constitutes a polychrest. The classification is to some extent dependent upon the scale of the **provings** to which the substance has been submitted and the clinical experience of its use, and hence the progress in the development of its **materia medica**.
3 The following medicines are included in the group of polychrests cited in homeopathic literature, but the list is not universally accepted nor regarded as exhaustive: *Argenticum nitricum, Arnica, Arsenicum album, Belladonna, Bryonia, Calcarea carbonica, Calcarea phosphorica, Carbo vegetabilis, Gelsemium, Ignatia, Ipecac, Lachesis, Lycopodium, Natrum muriaticum, Nux vomica, Phosphous, Pulsatilla, Rhus toxicodendron, Sepia, Silicea, Sulphur, Thuja.*

Synonym: **major remedy**

See also: **frequently used remedies, small remedy, status of medicines**

Etymology: ML *polychrestus* f. Gk *polychrestos* useful for many purposes (*poly* + *chrestos* useful)

polypharmacy

● Pharmacy, Therapeutics
1 Multiple drug therapy.
2 The practice of preparing or prescribing medicines
   containing more than one medicinal substance, or of
   administering several different medicines at the same
   time or concurrently.

Comment:
Despite being frequently used, the practice is
deprecated in all forms of medicine, but particularly
unicist homeopathy.
See also: **complex homeopathy, pluralist homeopathy**
Etymology: Gk *polu-* (*polus* much, *polloi* many)

polypragmasy

● Therapeutics
Administration of a number of different therapeutic
agents or regimes concurrently.
See also: **pluralist homeopathy, polypharmacy**
Etymology: Gk *polu-* (*polus* much, *polloi* many) + *pragma*
act, deed

ponderal dose

See: **material dose**

ponderation

See: **weighting of symptoms**
Etymology: L *pondus* weight

portrait

See: **clinical picture, constitution, drug picture,
symptom picture, picture, typology**

posology

● Pharmacology and drug action, Pharmacy,
Therapeutics
The science of dose regimes; the study of the size and

frequency of doses; a branch of pharmacology and therapeutics concerned with determining the doses of medicines.

Comment:
Today the quantity as opposed to the dilution of a dose is regarded by most practitioners as of no importance, but **Hahnemann** prescribed definite quantities.

See also: **dosage form, dosage regime, dose**

Etymology: Gk *posos* how much + *-logia* subject of study (*logos* account, discourse)

potence

● Philosophy

An entity possessed of and capable of exerting power upon or within an organism, but which cannot be explained by physical causes or perceived by the senses.

Comment:
1 The word used by Hahnemann in the *Organon* is 'Potenz'. He uses the terms 'potence,' **'Wesen'** and 'agent' interchangeably. A potence can be healthful or harmful, natural or artificial. He first applied the term to the power of naturally occurring causative agents of **disease** ('inimical potences') and then to the 'artificial disease potences' or drug potences, the medicines which have the power to evoke a healing response to the disease.
2 '*Potenz*' is translated as **potency** when it refers to the result of the **potentisation** of a medicine. The two concepts need to be clearly distinguished.

Etymology: L *potentia* power

potency

● Biophysics and biochemistry, Pharmacology and drug action, Therapeutics
1 Power; ability to cause effects.
2 The medicinal power of a homeopathic medicine,

released or developed by **dynamisation** or **potentisation**.

3   The measure of the power of the medicine based on the degree to which it has been potentised, expressed in terms of the degree of **dilution** (see **potency scale**).

Comment:
The concept of potency needs to be clearly distinguished from the concept of **potence**.

See also: **bioenergetics, bioinformation, dilution, dynamis, fluxion, potency energy**

Etymology: L *potentia* power (*potens -entis* part. of *posse* to be able)

potency chord

See: **potency complex**

potency complex

● Pharmacy

A homeopathic prescription in which two or more potencies of the same medicine are combined in one dose form.

Synonym: **potency chord**

potency energy

● Biophysics and biochemistry, Pharmacology and drug action

The **bioenergetic** properties of a **potentised** medicine.

Comment:
One hypothesis of the action of homeopathic potencies is that they establish a resonance between the energy field of the medicine and the energy field of the patient. Hence the potency energy stimulates the **life force** of the patient, activating or reinforcing the healing process.

See also: **dynamis, dynamisation, information, vital force**

potency, high

● Pharmacology and drug action, Pharmacy

Commonly held to be **potencies** above the 30th **centesimal potency** (30c) (= 10^{-60}).

Comment:
This distinction is controversial and to some extent arbitrary. In France the term may be applied to 12c and above, but high potency is held by some teachers and practitioners to extend even down to 9c. The concept of high, **medium** and **low potency** is arbitrary. It can be of practical value in discussing the appropriate use of different potency ranges in different clinical states. The widespread use of high potencies is largely attributable to the influence of **Kent**.

See also: **potency low, potency medium, potency scale**

potency, low

● Pharmacology and drug action, Pharmacy

Potencies below the 24th **decimal** or 12th **centesimal potency** (10^{-24}).

Comment:
This distinction between high, medium and low potency is controversial and to some extent arbitrary. It can be of practical value in discussing the appropriate use of different potency ranges in different clinical states, but even low potencies can have the profound effects more usually associated with higher potencies if the medicine is the **simillimum**.

See also: **potency high, potency medium, potency scale**

potency, medium

● Pharmacology and drug action, Pharmacy

Medium potencies are considered to lie within the range 12–30c (**centesimal potency**) in most countries, although in France the limit may be lower.

Comment:
The concept of **high**, medium and **low** potency is

controversial and to some extent arbitrary. It can be of practical value in discussing the appropriate use of different potency ranges in different clinical states.

See also: **potency high, potency medium, potency scale**

potency scale

● Pharmacology and drug action, Pharmacy, Therapeutics

Scale denoting the measure or degree of potency of homeopathic medicines.

Illustrations of potencies on different scales

Potency abbreviation	Meaning
c	centesimal, understood to be Hahnemannian
cH, CH, C.H.	centesimal potency (Hahnemannian potency)
cK	Korsakov potency
200D	200th decimal potency (Dunham scale – historical)
D, DH	decimal potency (Hahnemannian potency)
F	fluxion potency
FC	fluxion centesimal potency
K	Korsakov potency
LM1–LM30	Hahnemannian LM potencies
M, 10M, 50M, CM, DM, MM	millesimal potencies 1:1000 dilution, usually Korsakovian or Hahnemannian followed by Korsakovian
MK	millesimal potency=10^3 (Korsakov potency)
MT, TM, Ø	mother tincture
Q1–Q30	Q (LM) potency
x (6x–60x)	decimal potency (Hahnemannian potency)

See separate entries for details of particular potency scales listed here.

potentisation

● Biophysics and biochemistry, Pharmacology and drug action, Pharmacy

A multi-step process developed by **Hahnemann** by which the medicinal power (**potency**) of a homeopathic medicine is released or increased, involving **serial dilution** with **succussion**, or using **trituration** or **fluxion**.

Comment:

1 The process of potentisation was developed as a consequence of Hahnemann's observation that the method of dilution with succussion which he introduced to reduce the adverse effects of the medicines in the material doses that he first used increased the therapeutic power of the medicine. Succussion is essential to this process.

2 There is ambiguity about the use of the terms 'potentisation' and 'dynamisation'. Potentisation implies the process of dilution as well as succussion. **Dynamisation** is commonly used as synonymous with potentisation, but contemporary practitioners sometimes apply the term to the process of succussing the potentised medicine between doses to increase the potency, with or without further dilution (see **plussing**). Hahnemann himself uses both terms in this latter sense in separate passages of the *Organon*.

See also: **potency energy**

potentised allopathics

See: **tautopathy**

powder

● Pharmacy

1 The raw material used for **trituration** during the manufacture of homeopathic medicines, usually **lactose**.

2 A triturated medicine.

3 A unit **dosage form** for administering a homeopathic medicine, made by impregnating lactose with a **liquid potency** or by the addition of a few medicated **granules** (globuli). Powders may be administered directly, in a capsule or dissolved in water.

4 A bulk dosage form.

practitioner

● Main category

1 One who puts into practice a particular skill or technique.

2 One who practises a therapeutic technique.

3 A member of a healthcare profession.

precipitating factor

● Case taking and analysis, Disease processes, Symptomatology

1 The factor that triggers a particular event or change in state.

2 The factor responsible for the **onset** of an **illness**, or an episode of illness, or that triggers a particular symptom.

Comment:
Must be distinguished from an **aggravating factor**, which results in an existing state becoming worse, and an **etiological factor** which is primarily responsible for the existence of the state made manifest by the precipitating factor. For example, flashing lights may precipitate convulsions or an episode of migraine, but are not their underlying cause.

Synonym: **provoking factor**

See also: **aggravation, causal factor, causation, causative, causality, modality, never well since, occasion, therapeutic aggravation**

Etymology: L *praecipitare* throw or cast headlong (pre- + *ceps, cipitis* f. *caput* head)

predisposition

- Disease processes, Healing processes

  A pre-existing tendency towards a certain state.

  See also: **constitution, disposition, heredity, terrain, trait**

prescribing strategy

- Therapeutics

  The planned choice of and possible sequence of medicines to be prescribed in a treatment regime, and the rationale for this.

  See also: **alternating remedies, classical homeopathy, complex homeopathy, differential diagnosis, unicist homeopathy, pluralist homeopathy, second prescription**

  Etymology: L *prae- scribere* to write, direct in writing

presentation

  See: **dosage form**

presenting problem

- Case taking and analysis, Symptomatology

  The **complaint** described by the patient at the first consultation for that problem.

  See also: **anamnesis, evaluation of symptoms**

  Etymology: L *praesentare* (*prae* + *esse* to be at hand)

preservation

- Pharmacy
1 Keeping safe; maintaining the integrity of something.
2 The use of a preservative to maintain the activity and quality of a **liquid potency**. This is usually achieved by combining alcohol with water as the **vehicle** in the **dilution** process. **Hahnemann** originally used charcoal before he developed alcoholic dilutions.

preventive treatment

● Therapeutics

Use of treatment to avoid (primary prevention), to stop or hinder the development of (secondary prevention), or to minimise the complications of (tertiary prevention) an **illness** or **disease process**.

Comment:
1 Homeopathic and **isopathic** medicines may be used to prevent illness or injury. Examples include the use of *Arnica* (indicated for trauma) before surgery, the isopathic use of **allergens** to prevent allergic reactions.
2 The use of homeopathic nosodes preventively in place of conventional **immunisation** has been advocated but there is no **evidence** that the method is effective.

Synonym: **prophylaxis** (primary prevention)
Etymology: L *prae* + *venire* to come, to come before

primary action

See: **primary drug action**

primary drug action

● Pharmacology and drug action, Therapeutics

The immediate impact of a drug on the organism. Thus, if the homeopathic medicine is the correct **simillimum** it will cause a transient **aggravation** of the existing symptoms through its own direct effect, though this may be imperceptible to the patient.

Synonyms: **initial action, primary action**
See also: **biphasic action, pharmacodynamics, secondary drug action, therapeutic aggravation**
Etymology: L *primus* first

professional homeopath

● Practitioner

Homeopathic **practitioner** who has undergone a prescribed and supervised course of instruction, but who is not medically qualified.

Comment:
The legal status of professional homeopaths varies from country to country. In some countries their practice is licensed and regulated (e.g. Heilpraktiker in Germany, homeopathic practitioners holding degrees such as BHMS, DHMS and LCEH in India, and Naturopathic Doctors (ND) in some US states); in others it is illegal; while in some such as the UK they are free to practise without regulation.

See also: **doctor, lay homeopath, non-medically-qualified practitioner, physician**

Etymology: L *professio* declaring publicly

prognosis

● Disease processes, Healing processes

The predicted course or outcome of an **illness**; either in respect of the **natural history** of the **disease process**, or following treatment.

Comment:
In homeopathy prognosis is not based on the existing **pathology** and the natural history of the disease process to the same extent as in conventional clinical practice. Factors such as the **vitality** of the patient and the nature and behaviour of previous or coexisting disorders will be of particular significance.

Etymology: Gk *prognosis* (*pro* before + *gignosko* to know)

prophylaxis

See: **preventive treatment** (primary prevention)

Etymology: Gk *pro-* before + *phulasso* a guard (*phulaxis* guarding)

prover

● Materia Medica, Pharmacology and drug action

Subject of a **proving**, or **homeopathic pathogenetic**

trial. A volunteer, who should be in good health, who records changes in his or her condition during and after the administration of the substance to be tested.

Comment:
The definition of what constitutes good health in this context is not generally agreed.

Synonym: **volunteer**

proving

- Drug action, History, Materia medica, Pharmacology, Therapeutics
1 Testing the qualities of something.
2 Demonstrating the truth of a proposition by evidence or argument.
3 The process of determining the medicinal properties of a substance; testing substances in **material dose**, **mother tincture** or **potency**, by administration to healthy volunteers, to elicit effects from which the therapeutic potential, or **materia medica** of the substance may be derived.
4 Effects of a homeopathic medicine used in treatment that are characteristic of the **materia medica** of the medicine itself and not of the patient or the illness.

Comment:
1 Term for **homeopathic pathogenetic trial**; an anglicisation of the German 'Prüfung' used by **Hahnemann** to denote homeopathic trials in healthy volunteers. Now considered obsolete by some.
2 It is arguable that a proving, as defined in **4** above, should be regarded as an **adverse drug reaction**, although it resolves without harm to the patient when the prescription is stopped.

Synonyms: **drug proving, experimental pathogenesis**

Etymology: Ger *Prüfung* test, examination (*klinische Prüfung* clinical trial)

proving symptoms

● Disease processes, Materia medica,
  Therapeutics

1 The symptoms recorded by the subjects of a
   homeopathic pathogenetic trial or **proving**,
   and that contribute to the development of the
   materia medica of the substance under
   investigation.

2 Symptoms experienced by patients that are the
   product of the homeopathic medicine with which they
   are being treated, and characteristic of its **materia
   medica**, rather than of the **disease process** itself or
   some other intercurrent event.

   See also: **adverse drug reaction, iatrogenic, new
   symptoms**

provoking factor

   See: **precipitating factor**

pseudo-psora

   See: **tubercular diathesis**

psora

   See: **psoric miasm**

psoric miasm

● Disease processes, Materia Medica, Philosophy,
  Therapeutics

   Susceptibility to or manifestation of a particular
   pattern of **morbidity** originally associated with
   itching skin eruption; more recently associated
   with a pattern of disorder characterised by
   underreaction of the organism's self-regulating
   mechanisms. One of the three chronic **miasms**
   described by **Hahnemann**.

   Synonym: **psora**

   See also: **diathesis, itch diathesis**

   Etymology: Heb *tsorat* blemish, taint, dirt, stigma

psyche

● Philosophy, Symptomatology

Variously, the soul, the spirit, the mind; but in any case those attributes of the individual that are not of the physical body.

Etymology: Gk *psukhe* breath, soul, life

psychoneuroimmunology

● Disease processes, Healing processes, Physiology

The study of the interaction between emotional and other psychological states, the **neuropeptide** system and the **immune system**, affecting the individual's **susceptibility** or resistance to **illness** and **disease**.

Comment:

It is postulated that homeopathic medicines may in some cases act by influencing the chain of interaction between these systems, stabilising or supporting the immune response to psychological stress.

pulverisation

See: **grinding**

Etymology: LL *pulverizare* (*pulvis* dust)

q

Q potency

● Pharmacy

Alternative name for **LM potency** derived from the
Latin *quinquagintamillesima* (50 000); used because
the Roman numerals LM actually mean 950, not L (50)
x M (1000). Individual manufacturers use one or other
name according to preference.

Quin, Frederic Hervey Foster

● Biography

The first British homeopathic physician (1799–1878),
mistakenly believed to the son of the Duchess of
Devonshire whom he served as personal physician in
Italy from 1820–1824 where he was introduced to
homeopathy by **Neckar**, introduced homeopathy to
Italy and became physician to the Queen of Etruria in
Rome in 1824. Quin then became physician to Prince
Leopold, later King of the Belgians. He settled in
London in 1832, founded the **British Homoeopathic
Society** in 1844, and because of his aristocratic
connections was able to obtain the funds to establish
the **London Homoeopathic Hospital** in 1849. He was
physician to the household of Augusta, Duchess of
Cambridge and numbered other royalty among his
patients. His reputation as a wit and his friendship
with the Prince of Wales gave him social popularity

and entrée to all the great houses and ensured political support for homeopathy when needed.

quinine

Active principle of **Cinchona** officianalis

r

Rademacher, Johann Gottfried

● Biography

Proponent of **empirical medicine** (1772–1850), he
influenced homeopaths, reviving an interest in
organotherapy. He denied the law of the simile principle.

randomised controlled trial

● Clinical research

A clinical study which has three aspects of control:
(i) a comparative design with a treatment group that
acts as control; (ii) randomised allocation to treatment
groups in order to provide structural and
representational comparability; (iii) a protocol for its
conduct to provide observational comparability.
Etymology: OF *randon* at great speed (*randir* gallop)

ranking of symptoms

● Symptomatology, Therapeutics

The ordering of **symptoms** according to their
importance for **case analysis** or **repertorisation**.
See also: **evaluation of symptoms, hierarchy of
symptoms, weighting of symptoms**

rational

● Philosophy

1 Pertaining to reasoning or to the higher thought

processes; based on objective or scientific
knowledge.

2 Influenced by reasoning rather than by emotion.

3 Able to reason; endowed with reason; free from any
impairment of consciousness, thought disorder or
other condition which diminishes the capacity for
reasoning.

Etymology: L *rationalis* (ratio reason)

raw material

See: **source material**

reaction

● Physiology, Symptomatology

1 Response to a stimulus.

2 In homeopathy, a type of **general symptom** involving
the patient's reaction to environmental or psychosocial
factors.

See also: **aversion, desire, modality, reactivity,
response to the remedy**

Etymology: L *re-* again + *agere* act, do

reactivity

● Pharmacology and drug action, Physiology,
Therapeutics

The capacity of an organism to show a reaction to a
stimulus, including a drug stimulus.

Comment:
It is suggested that the reactivity of an organism to a
specific homeopathic medicine depends upon its
receptivity when in the particular disordered state to
which that medicine corresponds.

Etymology: L *re- again* + *agere* act, do

reappearance of old symptoms

● Case taking and analysis, Disease processes, Healing
processes

Symptoms which appear to have resolved in the past

but which recur temporarily in response to homeopathic treatment. Considered to indicate a favourable **prognosis** in homeopathy.

Comment:

1 The principles of the **direction of cure** include the observation that symptoms regress in the order in which they first appeared. This may involve the reappearance of old dormant symptoms which subsequently resolve as the healing process proceeds and more recent symptoms resolve in their turn.

2 This principle is accepted in varying degrees by different **schools**.

See also: **suppression, therapeutic aggravation**

receptivity

● Pharmacology and drug action, Physiology, Therapeutics

Ability to receive a stimulus.

Comment:

In homeopathy, it is evidently the disordered state of the organism, expressed by the symptomatology, that makes it receptive to the action of the **simillimum**, the medicine which corresponds to that **symptom picture**. This renders the organism sensitive to the precisely corresponding homeopathic prescription.

See also: **reactivity**

Etymology: ML *receptivus* able to receive f. L *re-* + *capere* to take

recovery

● Healing process

1 Process by which control is regained, or the ill effects of an event or situation are no longer felt.

2 The restoration of **health** after an **illness**.

3 In homeopathy, the process by which the functional equilibrium of the patient is restored or improved

by the action of the **life force** and
autoregulation.

See also: **cure, entelechy, healing**

Etymology: L *recuperare* recover

reductionism

● Medical methods, Philosophy

The view that systems can be analysed and understood
in terms of their separate component parts; that a
complex concept or system can be reduced to
its separate elements, rather than understood as a
whole.

See also: **holism, mechanistic**

Etymology: L *re-* + *ducere* to bring

relationship of remedies

● Materia medica, Pharmacy, Therapeutics

The interactive relationship of different homeopathic
medicines which may have beneficial or detrimental
effects.

See also: **antidote, complementary remedy,
concordances, following remedy, inimical,
synergism**

remedies that follow well

See: **following remedy**

remedy

● Healing processes, Pharmacy, Philosophy,
Therapeutics

1 The means of removing or improving any undesirable
state.

2 The means of curing or relieving a **symptom** or
disease.

3 The term commonly and colloquially used amongst
homeopaths for the homeopathic medicine because it
implies both the more comprehensive remedial action
which the prescription is expected to achieve and the

more purposive relationship to what is to be remedied in the patient than the more general term 'medicine'. Medicine is, however, the preferred term in this dictionary.

See also: **cure, drug, homeopathic medicine**

Etymology: L *re-* + *mederi* to heal

remedy picture

See: **drug picture**

remedy reaction

See: **response to prescription**

repertory

● Materia Medica, Symptomatology

1 Systematic cross reference of **symptoms** and **disorders** to the homeopathic medicines in whose therapeutic repertoire (**materia medica**) they occur. The strength or degree of the association between the two is indicated by the type in which the medicine name is printed.

2 Source used in case analysis to identify the medicine **indicated** for the patient. This process is called **repertorisation**.

Comment:

1 Data from the therapeutic repertoire of medicines appearing in the repertories are not always found in the materia medica, and vice versa, and the validity of data in the repertories is not always proven.

2 Both printed and electronic versions of repertories now exist.

See also: **rubric, weighting of symptoms**

Etymology: LL *repertorium* f. L *reperire* to find

repertorisation

● Case taking and analysis, Therapeutics

1 Use of **repertory** for decision support in homeopathic **case analysis** and prescribing.

2 The technique of using a repertory to identify the homeopathic medicines whose **materia medica** corresponds most closely to the **clinical picture** of the patient and from amongst which the **simillimum** may be chosen.

Comment:
1 Repertorisation cannot be depended upon alone to identify the best prescription. It can only suggest possible choices. The prescriber's knowledge of the patient and the materia medica must ultimately determine the choice.
2 This hitherto laborious process is now made easier and greatly enhanced by the development of computerised repertorisation systems.

See also: **evaluation of symptoms**

repetition of the dose

● Case taking and analysis, Therapeutics
1 Principles governing the dosage regime for homeopathic medicines.
2 The judgement of when to repeat a dose of a remedy to which a patient is responding.

Comment:
Regimes for the administration of homeopathic medicines vary from fixed schedules of regular dose repetition over a period of time to completely flexible regimes based on careful review of the patient's progress.

See also: **classical homeopathy, dosage regime, dose, posology, response to prescription, second prescription, single dose, unicist homeopathy**

response to prescription

● Case taking and analysis, Disease processes, Healing processes, Therapeutics

The changes in the patient's state which follow the administration of the homeopathic medicine and which cannot be accounted for by the natural history of the disease or intercurrent events.

Comment:
These observations require the same diligent attention to detail as the original **case taking** and **case analysis**, on which successful treatment depends. **Kent** describes 12 observations of the response to the prescription on which the **prognosis** may be based in his *Lectures on Homoeopathic Philosophy*. The contemporary Greek homeopath George Vithoulkas describes 27 such reactions in his *Science of Homeopathy*.

Synonym: **remedy reaction**

See also: **adverse drug reaction, direction of cure, obstacle to cure, reactivity, second prescription, pathography, prognosis, sensitive type**

revitalising

See: **plussing**

risk

● Therapeutics

1   The chance or probability that an unwanted event will occur; exposure to such mischance or hazard.
2   In medicine, any hazard or danger associated with medical treatment or related procedures; including **adverse drug reactions**, hazards associated with diagnostic procedures, and those associated with any **therapeutic encounter** or intervention, including the giving of advice and other aspects of the therapeutic encounter.

Medical risk is classified as direct and indirect. Direct risk arises from the direct effect of the medication or other intervention itself. Indirect risk comprises dangers arising, not from the medication or intervention, but from procedures, practices and beliefs associated with it.

Comment:
The direct risks of homeopathy appear to be slight; but where its practice is unregulated there is a greater

possibility of indirect risk arising from advice given by
practitioners who lack appropriate training or ethical
standards.

route of administration

● Therapeutics

The route by which the medicine enters the body. Most
commonly oral, usually dissolved in the mouth but
also swallowed. Also by inhalation, injection,
application and rectally. The intravenous route is rarely
used for homeopathic medicines. Administration of
the medicine via the breast milk after giving the dose
to the mother was the route recommended by
Hahnemann for the nursing infant, and is still
employed today. He also recommended rubbing the
medicine into the skin in addition to the oral route for
the cure of old diseases. These latter two routes are
now rarely used.

See also: **administration of the medicine, dosage
form**

Royal London Homoeopathic Hospital

See: **London Homoeopathic Hospital**

rubric

● Case taking and analysis, Materia Medica,
Symptomatology

1   The heading of a section of a document written in
distinctive print (traditionally red).

2   The phrase used in a **repertory** to identify a **symptom**
or **disorder** and its component elements and details,
and categories of these, and to which a list of the
medicines which are known to have produced that
symptom or disorder in **homeopathic pathogenetic
trials,** or to have remedied it in clinical practice, is
attached.

Etymology: L *rubrica* (*ruber*) red

S

saccharum album

See: **sucrose**

Etymology: Gk *sakkharon* sugar, L *albus* white

sarcode

● Drug action, Pharmacology, Pharmacy, Therapeutics

1 Historical term for the protoplasm of protozoa before the term protoplasm was introduced.
2 Homeopathic medicine derived from healthy human, animal tissue or organ.

See also: **isopathy, nosode, organotherapy**

Etymology: Gk *sarx, sark-* flesh + *eidos* resembling

scarlet fever

● Disease processes, History

An acute infectious exanthematous disease with characteristic rash caused by strains of group A, β hemolytic streptococcus producing erythrogenic (literally 'red-making') toxin. The bacterium was first isolated from the blood of scarlet fever patients by Klein in 1887. It was a common **epidemic disease** in Hahnemann's day, and a major cause of death, especially among infants. Hahnemann introduced *Belladonna*, whose toxic effects resemble scarlet fever, as a treatment and prophylactic for the disease in 1801 with great success. He was severely criticised for announcing that he would disclose his discovery only on payment of a fee of one gold piece from 300 contributors. He later relented. Scarlet fever was first described by **Sydenham**, a fact acknowledged in the *Organon*.

See also: **epidemic diseases, epidemic remedy**

Schmidt, Pierre

● Biography

Influential Swiss homeopathic physician (1894–1987). He studied with **Kent** and translated the *Organon* and other works of **Hahnemann** into French.

school

● Medical methods, Philosophy, Therapeutics

In homeopathy, a tradition of **philosophy** or therapeutics teaching a distinctive **doctrine**; may be named according to the method taught (e.g. **pluralist**, **unicist**, **classical**) or after the teacher who pioneered the doctrine (e.g. **Kentian**).

Schüssler, Wilhelm Hendrich

● Biography

German physician (1821–1898), originator of **biochemic medicine** and the Schüssler salts. He was greatly influenced by Virchow's theory of cellular pathology, which asserted that all disease processes originated in abnormalities in the cells. Although he prepared his medicines by **dynamisation** to **low potency** (6x), he was one of a number of homeopaths who were determined to reconcile the principles of homeopathy with conventional pathology. Despite entitling his original work on the tissue salts *An Abridged Homeopathic Therapeutics*, he later denied any connection with homeopathy.

Schüssler remedies

See: **biochemic medicine**

Schüssler salts

See: **biochemic medicine**

second prescription

● Therapeutics

The next medicine to be prescribed following the
original homeopathic prescription.

Comment:
The choice and timing of the second prescription is an
important aspect of the homeopathic therapeutic art.
Although some regimes involve regular repetition of
the dose, it may be necessary to wait patiently,
sometimes for weeks or even months, while the
response to the first prescription proceeds. The
decision to prescribe again, whether a **repetition of
the dose**, a change of **potency** or a different medicine,
must be based on positive **indications** that such a
course is necessary.
See also: **following remedy, repetition of dose,
response to prescription, single dose, unicist
homeopathy**

secondary drug action

● Pharmacology and drug action

Second phase of the response to the homeopathic
medicine. The phase that begins to show the healing
effect of the medicine, in contrast to the **therapeutic
aggravation** that may accompany the **primary drug
action**.
See also: **counteraction, dose-dependent reverse
effect, taxic drug action**
Etymology: L *secundus* following

self-healing

● Physiology

The natural capacity of an organism for **homeostasis**,
self-regulation (**autoregulation**) and **healing**.

self-regulation

> *See:* **autoregulation**

semiotics

- Symptomatology
1 Synonym for **symptomatology**.
2 In the context of linguistics, the study of signs and symbols.
  Etymology: Gk *semeiotikos* of signs (*semeion* sign)

sensation 'as if'

> *See:* **'as if' symptom**

sensitisation

- Physiology
  The process of being made sensitive or abnormally sensitive.
  See also: **receptivity**

sensitive patient

> *See:* **sensitive type**

sensitive type

- Case taking and analysis, Symptomatology, Therapeutics
1 Patient who shows unusual **reactivity** or responsiveness to a stimulus.
2 Individual who is particularly sensitive to a homeopathic medicine, or medicines.

  Comment:
  Such patients can experience an excessive response to repeated doses of homeopathic medicines.
  See also: **adverse drug reaction, constitution, receptivity, typology**

sensitivity

- Physiology
1 The ability to detect or recognise a particular stimulus.

2 A developed, possibly heightened, but not abnormal degree of responsiveness to a stimulus, or experience.

See also: **hypersensitivity, receptivity**

Etymology: L *sensitivus* (*sentire* to feel)

serial dilution

● Pharmacology and drug action, Pharmacy

A sequence of separate and equal **dilutions** from the same **stock**, each accompanied by **succussion** or **trituration**, comprising the separate **steps** in the **potentisation** of a homeopathic medicine.

See also: **centesimal potency, decimal potency, Hahnemannian potency, Korsakov potency, LM potency**

Etymology: L *series* row, chain (*serere* to join)

side-effects

See: **adverse drug reaction**

sidedness

See: **laterality**

sign

● Case taking and analysis, Symptomatology

Objective evidence or observation of the clinical state of the patient; objective evidence of disorder.

Comment:
In homeopathy, following **Hahnemann**'s interchangeable use of the terms symptom and sign for both subjective and objective manifestations of disorder, the term **symptom** is often used to refer to signs.

See also: **functional symptom, symptom picture**

Etymology: L *signum* mark, token

signatures, doctrine of

● Philosophy, Therapeutics

Symbolic parallels and correspondences between
nature and disease processes. A **doctrine** which
attributes therapeutic properties to plants on the
basis of some correspondence between their
characteristics (e.g. form, colour) and the
characteristics of the **disease** or the afflicted organ.
For example, the likeness of the *Euphrasia officianalis*
flower to a blue eye was believed to indicate its value
in eye diseases. This doctrine has been a part of
medical folklore for all time, but its most famous
exponent was the physician **Paracelsus** (1493–1542).
Mistakenly regarded as identical with the **similia
principle**.

See also: **anthroposophical medicine**

Etymology: LL *signatura* marking of sheep f. L *signare* to
mark

similar

● Case taking and analysis, Therapeutics

Drug picture similar to the **clinical picture**.

Comment:
There are different uses of the concepts **simile**
and **simillimum**. The terms may be used
synonymously, but 'similar' and 'simile' are also
used to describe a likeness between the drug picture
and the clinical picture which is not as precise as
the **simillimum**, and which may evoke a
response, possibly an **aggravation**, that does not
lead to therapeutic change. The equivalence or
difference of the concepts remains a matter for
debate.

See also: **similia principle**

Etymology: L *similis* like

similarity

See: **similia principle**

simile

See: **similar**

simile principle

See: **similia principle**

similia principle

● Philosophy, Therapeutics

The fundamental principle of **homeopathy**, which states that substances may be used to treat disorders whose manifestations are similar to those which they will themselves induce in a healthy subject. Expressed as *similia similibus curentur* (let like be cured by like).

Comment:

1 The concept that diseases could be eliminated by the medicinal use of substances which produced the same symptoms originated with **Hippocrates**. **Paracelsus** and other physicians later described the same phenomenon. Consequently **Hahnemann** effectively only rediscovered the principle during his **cinchona bark experiment** in 1790. He was the first physician, however, to investigate and develop it systematically.

2 The term 'law of similars' is used synonymously with similia principle, but the latter is preferred because the principle cannot be regarded as an established law in the same sense as, say, the physical laws of thermodynamics.

See also: **cinchona, similar, simillimum**

similia similibus curentur

● History, Philosophy

Latin phrase meaning 'let like be cured by like'. It expresses the fundamental principle of homeopathy, the **similia principle**. Sometimes incorrectly rendered as similia similibus *curantur* (like will be cured by like).

See also: **contraria contrariis curentur**

Etymology: L *similis* like

simillimum

● Case taking and analysis, Materia medica, Philosophy, Symptomatology, Therapeutics

The **drug picture** *most like* the **clinical picture** in the patient; the most accurate match between clinical **characteristics** of the patient and the **materia medica**; the basis of accurate and effective prescribing in homeopathy.

Comment:

The concept of the simillimum must be regarded as an abstraction because it is impossible to be absolutely sure that the chosen homeopathic medicine does have the drug picture most like the clinical picture in the patient. Prescribers will often choose a **similar**, one of possibly a number of medicines whose picture is very close to that of the patient but not the perfect simillimum, on the basis of their own current knowledge and ability, and according to the current sum of our knowledge of homeopathic medicines.

See also: **clinical picture, drug picture, totality of symptoms**

Etymology: L *similis* like *similimus* most like

Simmons, George Henry

● Biography

Influential American physician (1852–1937), born in England. He trained originally at the Hahnemann Medical College in Chicago and practised as a homeopath, but subsequently renounced homeopathy and trained at a conventional medical college. As General Secretary and General Manager of the American Medical Association for 12 years (1899–1911), and editor of its *Journal* for 25, he achieved far-reaching changes in the ethical, academic, scientific and professional standards of conventional medicine in America, all of which worked to the disadvantage of homeopathy. He was the driving force behind the **Flexner Report** which effectively led to the demise of homeopathic medicine in the USA.

simple substance

See: **life force**

single dose

● Therapeutics

The principle of administering only one **dose** of a single medicine derived from one **source material** at any one time; further doses being dependent on the principles governing the **repetition of the dose** and the **second prescription**. This is the basis of **unicist** homeopathy; often associated with the title of **classical homeopathy**.

See also: **complex homeopathy, pluralist homeopathy**

single flask method

See: **single glass method**

single glass method

● Pharmacy

Method of producing **serial dilutions** using the same single glass vial.

Comment:
Hering was the first to use the single glass method experimentally to manufacture homeopathic **potencies**, but he did not recommend this procedure. A few years later, in 1831 von **Korsakov** introduced this simplified potentising method to homeopathy. **Fluxion** potentisation is a special type of single glass method.

Synonym: **single flask method**
See also: **Korsakov potency, multiglass method**

single remedy

See: **single dose**

small remedy

See: **minor remedy**

solute

● Biophysics and biochemistry, Pharmacy

The substance dissolved in a solution. In homeopathic pharmacy the source of the liquid **potency**.

Etymology: L *solvere, solutus* unfasten(ed), free(d), release(d)

solution

● Biophysics and biochemistry, Pharmacology and drug action, Pharmacy

A liquid in which a solid or gas is dissolved.

Etymology: L *solvere, solutus* unfasten(ed), free(d), release(d)

solvation structures

● Biophysics and biochemistry

A hypothetical rearrangement of molecular structures in water and water–ethanol mixtures resulting from the process of **potentisation**. It is an extrapolation of the phenomenon of **clathrate** formation. The new arrangement is postulated as specific to the nature of the solute and the stage in the potentisation process.

See also: **cluster**

Etymology: L *solvere, solutus* unfasten(ed), free(d), release(d)

solvent

● Biophysics and biochemistry, Pharmacology and drug action, Pharmacy

Liquid used to produce a solution of a solid or gas.

See also: **solute, solution**

Etymology: L *solvere, solutus* unfasten(ed), free(d), release(d)

source material

● Materia medica, Pharmacology and drug action, Pharmacy

The original material from which the homeopathic medicines are prepared, and from which their therapeutic properties are derived; may be of botanical, chemical, mineral, human or animal origin, including pathological and microbiological materials. More unusual immaterial sources such as sunlight, X-rays and magnetism (**imponderabilia**) are also used.

Synonyms: **basic product, crude material, crude substance, raw material, starting material**

See also: **mother tincture, standardisation of drugs, stock**

specific

● Materia medica, Therapeutics
1 Definite; distinctive.
2 Appertaining to the characteristics of a species.
3 A homeopathic medicine specifically indicated for a particular clinical condition.

Comment:
There are few homeopathic specifics because the individual clinical picture is rarely so similar in all patients with a particular condition as to indicate one medicine, and some homeopaths deny that any true specific exists. The indication of *Arnica montana* for acute soft tissue trauma is a familiar example of a specific.

See also: **pathological prescribing**

Etymology: LL *specificus* f. L *species* appearance, kind (*specere* to look) + *facere* to make

specific effects

● Research, Therapeutics

The direct effects of a specific therapeutic intervention, as opposed to **non-specific effects**.

See also: **effectiveness, efficacy, placebo**

specifism

● Medical methods, Philosophy, Therapeutics

Therapeutic method based on the administration of homeopathic medicines chosen on the basis of **nosological** diagnosis or simply from the **tissue affinity** or **organ affinity**. This does not take into consideration the individual reactivity of the patient and should not be considered as truly homeopathic.

See also: **pathological prescribing, specific**

Etymology: LL *specificus* f. L *species* appearance, kind (*specere* to look) + *facere* to make

stability of medicines

● Pharmacology and drug action, Pharmacy

The maintenance of the properties of a medicine in a stable state.

Comment:

1 The maintenance of a stable state is essential if a medicine or its **source material** are to meet required pharmaceutical standards and fulfil expectations of **efficacy**.

2 Stability is difficult to confirm when the active properties are uncertain and not easily susceptible of measurement, as is the case with homeopathic **potencies**.

3 **Hahnemann** estimated stability of 18–20 years for homeopathic medicines from his observations, if protected from heat and light. Far greater periods of stability have been estimated since, as much as 140 years.

4 **Low potencies**, and especially **mother tinctures**, have limited stability because of their chemical ingredients, but it is believed that **high potencies** may be infinitely stable.

5 The French homeopathic **pharmacopeia** specifies that source materials must be renewed every five years, and also specifies the shelflife of **potencies** (usually also five years).

See also: **destruction of potency**

Etymology: L *stabilis* (*stare* stand)

standardisation of drugs

● Pharmacology and drug action, Pharmacy

The application of standard criteria to the properties of the **source material** and the method of preparation of medicines.

Comment:
Standardisation is a problem in homeopathic **pharmacy**. Although the French and German pharmacopeias regulate the nature and quality of the source material in detail, and the European pharmacopeia currently in preparation will do so, others do not, and there are few absolute criteria for identifying and monitoring their essential components and properties. On the other hand, methods of preparation of the medicines are strictly standardised in the various **pharmacopeias**, although methods of **succussion** are not.

Stapf, Johann Ernst

● Biography

German physician (1788–1860). The first physician to embrace homeopathy (1811), and a staunch friend and supporter of **Hahnemann**. He was a **prover** for the *Materia Medica Pura*. Hahnemann announced his **psora** theory to him and Dr. Gross in 1827. He achieved great fame as a clinician, so much so that in 1835 he was called to Britain to treat Queen Adelaide.

status of medicines

● Materia medica, Therapeutics

The importance of homeopathic medicines in respect of the extent of their therapeutic repertoire rather than their importance in the individual patient. This status is described in terms of their role as polychrests, frequently used remedies, major or minor remedies or small remedies.

Comment:
These 'status' terms are often a reflection of the extent or limitation of our knowledge of the **materia medica** rather than an absolute measure of the actual therapeutic repertoire.

Etymology: L *stare* stand

Steiner, Rudolph

- Biography
  Austrian philosopher and mystic (1861–1925) who founded **Anthroposophical medicine**.

step

- Pharmacology and drug action, Pharmacy
1 A **potency** level.
2 The separate stage in the sequence of **serial dilution** for preparation of a potency.
  Synonym: **lift in potency**
  See also: **dilution, dynamisation, potentisation**

stock

- Pharmacology and drug action, Pharmacy
  Substance or preparation used as starting material for **dilution** or **trituration** in the preparation of homeopathic **potencies**; may be the **source material** itself, or a **mother tincture** or **macerate**.
  Etymology: OE *stoc* trunk

strange, rare and peculiar symptom

- Case taking and analysis, Symptomatology
  Symptom that is highly **individual** because it is uncommon, surprising (e.g. **paradoxical**) or unusual in itself (e.g. a small child craving hot curry), idiosyncratic, or strikingly uncharacteristic of the **complaint** (such as a painless wound); of particular

significance in **case analysis** because of their highly individual nature, both in the patient and in the **drug picture** to which they correspond.

See also: **evaluation of symptoms, peculiar, symptom selection, weighting of symptoms**

subjective

● Case taking and analysis, Symptomatology

The individual description or interpretation of things perceived or experienced.

Comment:

The importance of the **individuality** of the **clinical picture** in homeopathic **case study** means that particular significance is attached to the subjective account of the illness, feelings and sensations, especially **as if symptoms**, and **modalities** and other particular **characteristic** somatic or mental symptoms. This is in contrast to the conventional approach which tends to attach greater importance to **objective** observations, although these also have a role in homeopathic **case taking** and analysis.

See also: **empirical**

substantial dose

See: **material dose**

succussion

● Biophysics and biochemistry, Pharmacology and drug action, Pharmacy

1 Shaking the body to detect the sound of fluid in a cavity.
2 Vigorous shaking, with impact or 'elastic collision', carried out at each stage of **dilution** in the preparation of a homeopathic **potency**.
3 One method of **potentisation**. The others are **fluxion** and **trituration**.

Comment:

Hahnemann is thought to have developed the process of succussion progressively over a number of years in the course of experimenting with different methods for diluting his medicines. He observed that the process enhanced the effectiveness of the medicine. The method of succussion and the rate, amplitude and number of succussions used in potentisation is not standardised, and varies between manufacturers. Within each manufacturing process, however, the number of succussions remains constant.

Etymology: L *sub-* under, close to, towards + *cutere*, *cussus* shake

sucrose

- Pharmacology and drug action, Pharmacy
1   Sugar obtained from sugarbeet and sugarcane; $C_{12}H_{22}O_{11}$.
2   A constituent of solid **dosage forms** and syrups.

See also: **lactose**

Etymology: F *sucre* sugar f. ML *succarum* f. Arabic *sukkar*

sugar

See: **sucrose**

sulphuric constitution

- Constitution, morphology and terrain

An elaboration by Henri **Bernard** of **Nebel**'s morphological types. Characteristically of moderate height and weight, balanced proportions and normal development.

Synonym: **normolinear constitution**

See also: **constitution, carbonic constitution, fluoric constitution, morphology, phosphoric constitution, typology**

suppression

- Disease processes, Symptomatology, Therapeutics

The **palliative** treatment of a symptom or condition so that it is relieved but is not resolved. It may remain dormant, or become manifest in some other, possibly more serious or deep-seated disorder.

Comment:

1 This is believed by homeopaths to be a common consequence of conventional **allopathic** and **antipathic** treatment. It may make subsequent homeopathic treatment more difficult, and needs to be recognised as part of the **pathogenesis** of the case so that an appropriate **prescribing strategy** can be planned.

2 Some homeopaths believe that suppression can also be induced by poor homeopathic treatment, but there is no general agreement about this.

See also: **direction of cure, reappearance of old symptoms, syndrome shift, vicariation**

Etymology: L *sub-* under + *primere* press

surrogate

● Materia medica, Therapeutics

1 Substitute.

2 Medicine used in the place of another, as an alternative for the same condition.

Comment:

Homeopathic teaching, and the concept of **individualisation** do not permit the possibility of surrogates. No two **source materials** have the same characteristics, and hence no two medicines have the same properties. Thus only one medicine can be the **simillimum** for the individual patient.

See also: **similar**

Etymology: L *sub-* under, close to, towards + *rogare* to ask

susceptibility

● Disease processes

1 Extent to which a person is receptive or open to influences; the manner in which and the degree to which a person is affected by outside influences.

2   Lack of resistance to harmful influence.
3   Vulnerability to illness.

Comment:
Perceiving the nature of a patient's susceptibility to illness is fundamental to the homeopathic approach. It is this susceptibility as well as the manifestation of the illness which homeopathic treatment seeks to address.
See also: **constitution, reactivity, receptivity, terrain**
Etymology: L *sub-* under, close to, towards + *capere* to take

suspension

● Pharmacy

A liquid form containing undissolved particles held suspended within the liquid.
See also: **colloid**
Etymology: L *sub-* under, close to, towards + *pendere* to hang

Swedenborg, Emanuel

● Biography, History, Philosophy

Swedish mathematician, scientist, inventor, mystic and theologian (1688–1772). At the age of 55 he abandoned science in favour of his own particular theology. His spiritual insights led him to deny orthodox trinitarian theology and proclaim Jesus as the single aspect of God. He believed that every material phenomenon had a spiritual counterpart. A protestant sect based on his teachings was founded in London in 1788. Several leading American homeopaths, most notably **Kent** and **Boericke**, were Swedenborgians.

sycosis

See: **sycotic miasm**

sycotic miasm

● Disease processes

A pattern of disorder originally attributed by

Hahnemann to the effects of gonorrhea and figwarts. Subsequently characterised by overreaction, overactivity or excess of body structure or function.

Synonym: **sycosis**

See also: **diathesis, miasm, psoric miasm, pseudo-psora, syphilitic miasm, tubercular diathesis**

Etymology: Gk *sukon* fig + *osis* forming

Sydenham, Thomas

● Biography

English physician (1624–89) who gave priority to observation in medicine and the avoidance of speculation. He was admired by **Hahnemann** because of this. His work anticipates many of the principles of homeopathy. For example, his clinical method was based on minutely detailed observation of the patient; 'his determination to observe and examine each individual patient with the open mind of a natural historian', and to 'listen intently and question the patient minutely about the march of events in the development of disease.' He regarded the manifestation of disease as 'an effort of nature, who strives with might and main to restore the health of the patient by the elimination of morbific matter.' (Marinker 1987) It is also notable that Sydenham adopted quinine (**cinchona**) for the treatment of ague (malaria). Hahnemann's curiosity about quinine, aroused by a monograph by **Cullen**, led to the experiment which was his first practical demonstration of the homeopathic principle.

symptom

● Case taking and analysis, Symptomatology

1 Any unexpected change in the normal state of mind or body experienced by the patient.

2 The term is sometimes also used in homeopathy to describe all the observed characteristics of the illness,

subjective and objective, expressed by the patient, observed by others or by the practitioner.

See also: **anamnesis, case taking, complete symptom, functional symptom, general symptom, local symptom, mental symptom, particular symptom, modality, totality of symptoms**

Etymology: Gk *sumptoma* chance (*sun* with, together + *pipto* fall, happen)

symptom picture

● Case taking and analysis

Description of the features of the **illness** in the individual patient. Virtually synonymous with **clinical picture**. Implies a **subjective**, patient-centred description, but usually includes **objective** observations of the clinician.

See also: **disease picture, symptom**

symptom selection

● Case taking and analysis, Therapeutics

The process of identifying those symptoms from the whole **clinical picture** of most value for homeopathic **case analysis** and the choice of the **simillimum**. Criteria applied to determine the importance of symptoms in this respect include:

◆ the spontaneity and vividness with which they are presented;
◆ the degree of emphasis given to them by the patient;
◆ their **individuality** to the patient as compared to their common association with the disease process;
◆ the **level** at which they affect the patient; the mental level often being held to be of particular importance;
◆ their strangeness, rareness or peculiarity.

Synonyms: **grading of symptoms, ranking of symptoms, ordering of symptoms, weighting of symptoms (ponderation)**

See also: **case taking and analysis, evaluation of symptoms**

symptomatology

● Symptomatology

1 The study and science of symptoms; their manifestation and behaviour, and their significance as **indications** of disease.
2 In homeopathy, the study of their value as indications for the homeopathic prescription.
3 The complete symptoms of a disease.

Comment:
In homeopathy symptoms are regarded as the expression of the organism's response to **disorder**, rather than its failure; just as in conventional physiology inflammation is known to be first and foremost a defence mechanism rather than a **disease process**.
See also: **case taking and analysis, materia medica, semiotics**
Etymology: symptom + Gk *-logia* subject of study (*logos* account, discourse)

syndrome

● Disease processes

The complex of **symptoms** and **signs** that represent a particular **disease process**. Not in itself precisely diagnostic of a particular pathology or cause, but descriptive of a group of related manifestations of disorder.
Etymology: Gk *sun-* with, together, alike *dramein* to run

syndrome shift

● Disease processes, Symptomatology

The phenomenon in which an existing **syndrome** is displaced by another; as when the symptoms of a pre-existing chronic illness are modified by an intercurrent acute illness.

Comment:
In homeopathy the concept has wider application. As well as the shift from one syndrome to another that is

observed in the **evolution** of the illness, alternation between syndromes is found to occur in many patients and to be a feature of a number of **drug pictures**. Also the shift of the focus of the illness from one system to another, or one **level** to another, which may occur during the response to treatment is an important feature of the case study.

See also: **alternating symptoms, direction of cure, layers of illness, level of illness, metastasis, suppression, vicariation**

synergism

● Pharmacology and drug action, Therapeutics

The combined or coordinated effect of separate processes which exceeds the effect of their individual actions. For example, the combined effect of different muscles in producing and controlling movement, or of different drugs in achieving better therapeutic effects. Certain combinations of homeopathic medicines are said to exhibit this effect.

Synonym: **Burgi's principle**

See also: **adjuvant, compatible, concordance**

Etymology: Gk *sun* together + *ergon* work

syphilitic miasm

● Disease processes

A pattern of chronic disorder originally attributed by **Hahnemann** to the effects of the venereal disease syphilis itself. Subsequently characterised by destructive change, breakdown or failure of body structure or function.

Synonyms: **destructive diathesis, lues, luetic miasm**

See also: **diathesis, miasm, psora, pseudo-psora, sycosis, tubercular miasm**

Etymology: mod L *Syphilus* name of a shepherd, portrayed as first sufferer from syphilis, in the poem of 1530 *Syphilis, sive Morbus Gallicus* (Syphilis or the French Disease) by Girolamo Fra-Verona.

system

● Philosophy

The integrated parts and functions of a complex entity; in this context a living organism.

See also: **model**

t

---

tautopathy

● Medical methods

Isopathic treatment with a **potentised** preparation of a chemical substance, especially a conventional drug, that has had or is having some adverse effect on the patient.

Comment:
Tautopathic medicines are prepared from about 150 conventional drugs (e.g. aspirin, chloramphenicol, diazepam, nitrazepam), industrial chemicals (e.g. solvents, paints), insecticides (e.g organophosphates, sheep dips) and household fluids (e.g. disinfectants, washing up liquids). The latter are often used for the isopathic treatment of allergies. Other uses of tautopathy are in the treatment of **adverse drug reactions**, **iatrogenic** disease, and possibly drug abuse. They are also useful in managing the withdrawal of conventional drug treatment.

Etymology: Gk *tauto, to auto* the same + *patheia* suffering

taxic drug action

● Pharmacology and drug action

The action of a drug in **dilution** which is the same as its action in a standard dose. For example, low **potencies** of estrogen exhibiting the same effects as a standard replacement dose in menopausal conditions.

See also: **antitaxic drug action**

temperature modality

● Symptomatology

The influence of temperature and changes in temperature on the behaviour of a symptom; including the local application of heat and cold to the affected part, the temperature of the immediate environment and the climate. Many homeopathic medicines include such symptom details in their **materia medica**.

See also: **general symptom, modality**

terrain

● Case taking and analysis, Constitution, morphology and terrain, Disease processes

1 The diverse characteristics of the individual that make him or her susceptible to **illness**. The 'soil' in which the 'seed' of the illness may be sown. The **susceptibility** of the individual **constitution**.

2 The living being, considered as a complete **system** in which **morphology**, anatomy, physiology, psychology, previous diseases and genetic inheritance make up the analytic factors of an indivisible whole.

See also: **typology**

Etymology: L *terrenus* of earth (*terra* earth)

Tessier, Jean-Paul

● Biography

Eminent member of the Paris school of homeopathy (1811–1862), who was influential in establishing homeopathy in France. He published prospective case series on pneumonia and cholera, and conducted large scale pragmatic trials of homeopathy vs allopathy.

theme

- Case taking and analysis, Philosophy, Symptomatology
1 The main subject or central idea of a discourse, narrative or musical composition.
2 In homeopathy, the characteristic or idea that runs through or links either the members of a group of related medicines (for example the 'weakness' in the **materia medica** of medicines derived from acids), or the different elements of a **case** (for example 'coldness' may be a feature of a patient's symptoms, body temperature and personality).

   Etymology: Gk *thema* place, proposition

   See also: **centre of the case, essence, family, Wesen**

therapeutic

- Therapeutics

   Curative, **healing**.

   Etymology: Gk *therapeutikos (therapeu* wait on, cure)

therapeutic aggravation

- Therapeutics

   Temporary worsening of existing symptoms following the administration of a correctly chosen homeopathic prescription, which indicates a favourable response to treatment.

   Comment:
   1 According to Hahnemann, in a therapeutic homeopathic aggravation a very similar medicinal disease displaces the patient's original disease. While it appears to the patient to be a worsening of pre-existing symptoms, it is actually the initial action (**primary drug action**) of the homeopathic medicine whose symptoms are somewhat stronger than those of the natural disease. In other words, the patient with a homeopathic aggravation is experiencing stronger medicinal symptoms, not his original disease symptoms.

2 Aggravations in response to homeopathic medicines can also occur when the chosen medicine is not the correct **simillimum**; for example, when the prescription is a close **similar** or **simile**. These reactions may involve symptoms that were not previously present in the patient and do not have the same favourable outcome as a therapeutic aggravation.

Synonym: **healing crisis, initial reaction, initial aggravation**

See also: **aggravation, complication, new symptoms, secondary drug action**

therapeutic encounter

● Therapeutics

The interaction between two or more people whose purpose is to improve the health or wellbeing of one or other or all of those involved.

Comment:

1 In a formal sense the therapeutic encounter is usually conceived in terms of the interaction between therapist and client, but it can be a group encounter. There may be more than one therapist or more than one client. The encounter may involve an explicit therapist–client (e.g. doctor–patient) relationship, or a mutually supportive relationship, as in co-counselling or a selfhelp group. Informal encounters in everyday life can, of course, also be therapeutic.

2 The effectiveness of the encounter will depend on its **non-specific effects**, as well as any specific therapeutic agent or technique employed.

3 The therapeutic effects of the **consultation** itself make an important contribution to the outcome of homeopathic treatment, irrespective of the **specific effects** or **efficacy** of the homeopathic medicine.

See also: **healing, placebo, therapeutic**

therapeutic modality

● Medical methods

The method employed in a therapeutic procedure; a

particular therapeutic approach. Homeopathy is a particular therapeutic modality.

See also: **biomedical model, therapeutic**

therapeutics

● Main category

The branch of medicine concerned with the practical treatment of disease or disorder; all aspects of the principles and methods of treatment.

Etymology: Gk *therapeutikos* (*therapeuo* wait on, cure)

therapy

● Therapeutics

The treatment of **disorder** or **disease**.

Etymology: Gk *therapeia* medical treatment, healing

thermal modality

See: **temperature modality**

time modality

● Symptomatology

The relation of symptoms and their behaviour to the time of day. Symptoms often show a characteristic time pattern or diurnal variation, occurring or remitting, worsening or ameliorating at particular times or over particular periods. Many homeopathic medicines include such symptom details in their **materia medica**.

See also: **general symptom, modality**

tincture

● Pharmacy, Therapeutics

1 A **solution** of a substance, often vegetable, used for medicinal purposes, in which alcohol, alcohol–water mixtures, water, glycerine or isotonic sodium chloride solution are used as a vehicle (**solvent**).

2 In homeopathic pharmacy this may comprise the
mother tincture, the **medicating potency,** or the
actual dosage form of the medicine in **potency.**
Etymology: L *tinctura* dyeing

tissue affinity

● Materia medica, Therapeutics

The tendency for a homeopathic medicine to act on a
particular type of body tissue. For example, the
medicine *Ruta* has a special affinity for fibrous tissue.
Synonym: **histiotropism**
See also: **affinity, disease affinity, organ affinity**
Etymology: OF *tissu* woven f. *tistre* (L *texere* weave)

tissue salts

● Medical methods

General title of the medicines used in **biochemic
medicine.**
See also: **Schüssler**
Etymology: OF *tissu* woven f. *tistre* (L *texere* weave)

tolerance

● Pharmacology and drug action, Therapeutics
1 The ability to bear or endure something.
2 The ability to take medicines without undesirable
effects or side-effects.
3 Progressive reduction in the patient's responsiveness to
a drug during long term medication. Hence the need
for increasing doses of a drug to achieve the same effect.
See also: **intolerance, reactivity, sensitivity**
Etymology: L *tolerare* to endure

totality of symptoms

● Case taking and analysis, Symptomatology

The complete **clinical picture** of the patient during
the **illness**; comprises all the **mental symptoms,
general symptoms** and **local (particular) symptoms**
and signs, and test findings if appropriate; the

complete symptom pattern from which the
simillimum must be found.

See also: **complete symptom, disease picture**

Etymology: L *totalis* (*totus* entire)

toxicity

⦿ Pharmacology and drug action, Pharmacy

The poisonous properties of substances, including
drugs.

Comment:
Many homeopathic medicines are derived from toxic
substances. In **low potency**, where the medicine
still contains a material dose of the toxic substance the
possibility of drug toxicity remains. Pharmaceutical
regulations prohibit the sale of low potencies
of homeopathic medicines derived from these
sources.

Etymology: Gk *toxa* arrows (*toxikon pharmakon* poison for
arrows).

toxicology

⦿ Materia Medica, Pharmacology and drug action,
Pharmacy

The study of the poisonous effects of substances; the
science of poisons, their source, composition, action,
identification, and **antidotes**. Source of much
homeopathic **materia medica**.

See also: **drug picture**

Etymology: Gk *toxa* arrows (*toxikon pharmakon* poison for
arrows) + *-logia* subject of study (*logos* account,
discourse)

toxin

⦿ Disease processes

1 Harmful or poisonous substance produced either as
an integral part of the cell or tissue, as a secretion, or
as a combination of the two, by certain
microorganisms and some plant and animal species.

2 Any chemical within the body whose accumulation is detrimental to health; may be introduced from outside the body (drugs, pollution), or produced within the body by the action of organisms, by the reaction of the body to circumstances (stress) or from **disease processes**.

See also: **antihomotoxic therapy, homotoxicology**

Etymology: Gk *toxa* arrows (*toxikon pharmakon* poison for arrows)

trait

● Case taking and analysis

1 Distinguishing feature of appearance or behaviour.
2 Characteristic aspect of an individual's personality, general **constitution** or family background.

See also: **constitution, diathesis, disposition, miasm, predisposition, susceptibility, terrain**

Etymology: L *tractus* drawing (*trahere* draw)

treatment

● Therapeutics

1 Procedure used in the care of a patient.
2 Any deliberately applied intervention for diagnostic, therapeutic or prognostic purposes in patient care, in a clinical study or as an intervention on a healthy subject in a pharmacological investigation.

See also: **intervention**

Etymology: OF *traitier* f. L *tractare* to handle (*trahere* to draw)

trial

See: **clinical trial**

Etymology: AF *trial, triel* (*trier* try)

trituration

● Pharmacy

1 Dilution in the solid phase, by **grinding**.
2 The first stages in the preparation and **potentisation**

of homeopathic medicines from solid and insoluble
source material, and in some cases from **fresh plants**,
by grinding it together with **lactose** as a **diluent**. In the
preparation of **liquid potencies** from triturations the
trituration may be dissolved in water to continue the
potentisation by **succussion**.

See also: **C3 trituration, dilution**

Etymology: L *triturare* thresh corn (*tritura* rubbing)

tubercular diathesis

● Case taking and analysis, Disease processes

1 A pattern of **morbidity** with features reminiscent of
the manifestations or sequelae of tuberculosis.

2 A pattern of morbidity that certain authors believe to
be linked to a hypothetical tubercular **toxin**.

Synonym: **pseudo-psora**

See also: **diathesis, miasm**

Etymology: L *tuberculum* diminutive of *tuber* lump

tuberculinism

See: **tubercular diathesis**

Tyler, Margaret Lucy

● Biography

Physician (1859–1943) who after some success as an
author qualified in medicine in 1903 at the age of 44.
Believing that British homeopathy did not follow the
tenets of **Hahnemann** she induced her parents to
establish scholarships to enable doctors to study under
Kent. She can be said to have been solely responsible
for the conversion of British homeopaths to **Kentian**
principles. She spent her whole medical career at the
London Homoeopathic Hospital. She lectured, ran a
correspondence course and edited the journal
Homoeopathy, which served as a textbook. She is best
known for her *Homoeopathic Drug Pictures*, published
in 1942.

See also: **drug pictures**

typhus

● Disease processes, History

A group of acute infectious and contagious diseases caused by microorganisms transmitted to humans by arthropods. Epidemic typhus is caused by *Rickettsia prowazekii* and spread by body lice; its spread is encouraged by crowded living conditions and poor personal hygiene. Endemic, or murine typhus is a milder form of epidemic typhus caused by *Rickettsia typhi* and transmitted to humans by rat or mouse fleas. The use of homeopathy in the typhus **epidemic** following Napoleon's retreat from Moscow in 1812–1813 was the first real demonstration of its **effectiveness**. Cases of typhus were successfully treated at the **London Homoeopathic Hospital** in 1891.

Etymology: Gk *tuphos* smoke, stupor

typology

● Case taking and analysis, Constitution, morphology and terrain

The study of characteristic patterns in the make up of patients; particularly their physique. Closely related to the concept of **constitution** and **terrain** in that it refers to the common characteristics of groups who show susceptibility to particular disorders and sensitivity to particular homeopathic medicines.

Comment:
In some uses typology lays more emphasis on physical shape (**morphology**) than other characteristics. In Italy and France, the constitution is also closely related to morphology.

Synonym: **drug type**

See also: **constitutional medicine, diathesis, fluoric constitution, Nebel, phosphoric constitution, sulphuric constitution**

Etymology: Gk *tupos* impression, figure, type

u

ultrahigh dilution

- Biophysics and biochemistry, Pharmacy

Substances in extreme **dilution** but which may have a
detectable molecular presence of the original matter.

Comment:
The term is sometimes used mistakenly in place of
ultramolecular dilution.

Etymology: L *ultra* beyond

ultramolecular dilution

- Biophysics and biochemistry, Pharmacology and drug
action

1 **Dilution** of a substance to the extent that no molecule
of the source material may be theoretically present in
the solution; the state of many homeopathic
potencies.

2 Dilution of a substance beyond **Avogadro's number**.

See also: **infinitesimal dose, ultrahigh dilution**

Etymology: L *ultra* beyond

unicist homeopathy

- Materia medica, Philosophy, Therapeutics

School or philosophy of homeopathic therapeutics
using a single homeopathic medicine at one time.

See also: **classical homeopathy, combination remedies, complex homeopathy, pluralist homeopathy, single dose, single remedy**

Etymology: L *unus* one

vaccination

● Therapeutics

The administration of a **vaccine**.

vaccine

● Therapeutics

A preparation used for **immunisation**. Originally the live cowpox virus inoculated into the skin to provide protection against smallpox.

See also: **immunisation, immunotherapy, vaccinosis**

Etymology: L *vaccinus* pertaining to the cow (*vacca cow*)

vaccinosis

● Disease processes

The syndrome produced by the adverse effects of vaccination; state of chronic ill health resulting from **immunisation**.

Comment:

1 The term was introduced in relation to the symptoms produced by smallpox vaccination in 1877 in a paper by a Dr Goullon of Weimar, but the concept was only fully developed by **Burnett** in the 1890s. The disorder is attributed to dysfunction of the immune system because it has been compromised rather than simply stimulated by immunisation.

2 The alleged adverse effects of immunisation are the cause of much controversy within homeopathy, although **Hahnemann** himself strongly favoured smallpox immunisation using the cowpox vaccine introduced by Edward Jenner in 1796, which he regarded as properly homeopathic.

See also: **immunisation, immunotherapy**

Etymology: L *vaccinus* pertaining to the cow (*vacca* cow)

Vannier, Leon

● Biography

Leading French homeopathic physician (1880–1963), very influential in his time. He was best known for his theories on typology.

Vegatest

● Biophysics and biochemistry, Medical methods

Technique which uses an instrument, a modified Wheatstone bridge (the Vega machine), claimed to be able to record the body's electrical energy passing through a circuit. An electrode held by the patient forms one end of the circuit, and another electrode, in the form of a stylus, applied by the practitioner to acupuncture points on the patient's hand or foot, the other. Substances are inserted into this circuit whose capacity to provoke or alleviate an adverse reaction is to be tested. The provocative agent and the correct medicine are believed to be identified by changes in the electrical current. This method is not part of mainstream homeopathy, but is used by some practitioners to select homeopathic medicines for the patient, usually **combination remedies**.

See also: **bioenergetics**

vehicle

● Pharmacy

1 The medium in which the medicine is presented.

2 The **diluent** used during the extraction of the active principles of plant materials, and in the **potentisation** process.

Comment:
The vehicle is generally considered to be inert. However there is evidence that the vehicle has an important role in assisting the way in which **potentisation** works and therefore could under some circumstances be considered as an **adjuvant**.

See also: **auxiliary substance, dosage form, excipient**

Etymology: L *vehiculum* (*vehere* carry)

veterinary homeopathy

● History

Homeopathic medicine has been used on animals since **Hahnemann**'s time. He delivered a lecture on the subject to the Leipzig Economic Society in c.1813, in which he outlined similar principles to those governing its use in humans. The practice of veterinary homeopathy was used extensively by **Boenninghausen** in the animals on his family estate. **Lux**, otherwise known as the father of **isopathy**, was another successful contemporary exponent and published his *Zooaiasis* (vol. 1) in 1832. Books on the subject abound from the 19th century, when the practice was widespread in the UK, US and Germany. In modern times there has been a renewal of interest. In 1982 the British Association of Homoeopathic Veterinary Surgeons was formed. In 1984 veterinary courses began at the **Royal London Homoeopathic Hospital**. In April 1986, the International Association for Veterinary Homeopathy was founded in Luxembourg. The first official veterinary qualification was awarded by the Faculty of Homoeopathy in 1987.

Comment:
In the UK, only statutorily registered veterinarians may treat animals, but no such protection applies to humans.

Etymology: L *veterinarius* (*veterinae* cattle)

vicariation

● Disease processes, Symptomatology

A description of the evolution of the disease process introduced by Reckeweg in his exposition of **homotoxicology**. It describes the transition of the disease process from one phase to a worse phase (e.g. eczema progressing to asthma) known as progressive vicariation, or to a better phase (e.g. asthma progressing to eczema) known as regressive vicariation.

See also: **alternating symptoms, direction of cure, metastasis, suppression, syndrome shift**

Etymology: L *vicarius* substitute (*vix vicis* change)

Vienna Provers' Union

● History

Full title 'Union of Austrian Homeopathic Physicians for Physiological Drug Proving'. Founded in 1842 it undertook and published many provings. In 1873 it became the Society of Homeopathic Physicians of Austria.

vis medicatrix naturae

● Philosophy
1 Healing power of nature.
2 The inherent ability of an organism to overcome disease and disorder and regain its health.

See also: **entelechy, healing, life force, vitalism**

vital force

See: **life force**

vitalism

● Philosophy

Philosophy that ascribes the origin of life in all living organisms to a vital principle that energises, sustains, directs and integrates their functions, which is distinct from any chemical or other physical principle. Closely related to the concept of the **life force** (vital force) which is a main theme of homeopathic philosophy.

See also: **autoregulation, bioenergy, dynamis, entelechy, healing**

Etymology: L *vita* life

vitality

● Healing processes

Liveliness. The state of being alive. Vital energy.

Etymology: L *vitalitas* (*vita* life)

volunteer

See: **prover**

weather modality

● Symptomatology

The effect of particular weather conditions or changes in weather on the behaviour of symptoms. Many homeopathic medicines include such symptom details in their **materia medica**.

See also: **modality, general symptom**

weighting of symptoms

● Case taking and analysis, Therapeutics

The measure of the differential importance of symptoms for the purposes of **case analysis** and selecting the homeopathic medicine. Symptoms are weighted on the basis of spontaneity (spontaneously reported by the patient rather than elicited on enquiry), clarity (clearly expressed by the patient), intensity (their severity or impact upon the patient), completeness (see **complete symptom**), and their peculiarity to the individual (see **strange, rare and peculiar symptoms**).

Synonym: **ponderation**

See also: **differential diagnosis, evaluation of symptoms, hierarchy of symptoms, repertory, repertorisation, symptom selection**

Weir, Sir John

● Biography

Scottish physician (1879–1971), one of the first to be

awarded a Tyler scholarship, he was a colleague of Margaret **Tyler** at the **London Homoeopathic Hospital**. He was the first homeopathic doctor to be appointed as Physician to the Royal Household, and his practice to royalty extended outside Great Britain.

wellbeing

● Healing processes, Therapeutics

A general sense of equanimity and satisfaction with oneself and one's life, an inner **vitality**, which may involve a positive acceptance of difficulty, disability or **disorder**, or other circumstances which adversely affect the individual. A state which leads a person to say 'I feel well in myself.'

Comment:
An increase in wellbeing is one of the most important signs of a good response to homeopathic treatment. It is often reported despite the occurrence of a **therapeutic aggravation** or the **reappearance of old symptoms**.
See also: **direction of cure, entelechy, healing, health, illness**

Wesen

● Philosophy
1   Essential quality of being, quintessence.
2   *Wesen* is a multifaceted German term which can mean any of the following: essence, substance, creature, living thing, nature, or entity. There is no single word in the English language that adequately translates *Wesen*.

Comment:
  1 In the ***Organon*, Hahnemann** uses the term in almost every instance to refer to that entity which is the essential unchanging *esse* of something: its being, its quintessence.
  2 A *Wesen* should not be regarded as an abstraction; it

is conceived as a dynamic, self-subsisting presence
which permeates the whole of something and is
indivisible from it, even though that presence is not
material and has no mass.

3 Hahnemann suggests that the *Wesen* of a **disease**
impinges upon the *Wesen* of the human being,
resulting in a particular set of **symptoms**. The
Wesen of a medicine is introduced in order to
retune the disturbed *Wesen* of the patient, thereby
restoring the patient to health. Hahnemann's use of
Wesen in these various contexts makes clear his
belief that the **life force**, diseases and medicines are
all operating in the same dynamic dimension.
(Hahnemann 1996 pp 361–363)

X Potency

See: **decimal potency**

References

British Medical Association 1993 Complementary medicine: new approaches to good practice. Oxford University Press, Oxford

Decker S (Translator) 1996 In: O'Reilly (Ed), Organon of the Medical Art. Hahnemann, S. Birdcage Books, Washington

Ernst E et al 1995 Complementary medicine – a definition. British Journal of General Practice 45:506

Gaier H 1991 Encyclopaedic Dictionary of Homoeopathy. Thorson's, London

Hahnemann, S 1996 Organon of the medical art. Ed: O'Reilly W B, Translator: Deckers. Birdcage Books, Washington

Koehler, G 1986 The handbook of Homoeopathy; its principles and practice. Thorsons, New York, p. 176

Marinker M 1987 The chameleon, the Judas goat and the cuckoo. Journal of the Royal College of General Practitioners 28: 199–206

Sackett D, Rosenberg W 1995 On the need for evidence-based medicine. Journal of the Royal Society of Medicine 88:602–604

Sources and Bibliography

Most of the definitions given here are original or composed from several sources. Those that owe their origin to one particular source are explicity referenced. Other sources used in compiling the dictionary are as follows:

British Homoeopathic Pharmacopoeia 1993 British Association of Homoeopathic Manufacturers, Derbyshire, Vol.1

Churchill's Medical Dictionary 1989 Churchill Livingstone, New York

Concise Oxford Dictionary 1982 Oxford University Press, Oxford

Dellmour F 1997 Homöopathie und Lebenskraft. Begriffe bei Samuel Hahnemann. Documenta Homoeopathica, Band 17, W. Maudrich, Wien

Dictionary of Chemistry 1988 Penguin, London

Dictionary of Epidemiology 1995 3rd edn, Last JM (ed). Oxford University Press, Oxford

Monograph on Homoeopathic Preparations 1999 European Pharmacopoeia Commission. 2000 supplement, p. 1038

German Homoeopathic Pharmacopoeia 1978 1st edn Translation of the German Homöopathisches Arzneibuch (HAB 1) Amtliche Ausgabe, Edited by British Homoeopathic Association. Deutscher Apothekerverlag, Stuttgart. Suppl. 1: 1981, Suppl. 2: 1983, Suppl. 3: 1985, Suppl. 4: 1985

Homöopathisches Arzneibuch (HAB 1) 1985 Amtliche Ausgabe, Deutscher Apothekerverlag Stuttgart, Govi-Verlag GmbH,

Frankfurt Enthält die Teilbande HAB 1 1978; 1. Nachtrag 1981; 2. Nachtrag 1983; 3. Nachtrag 1983; 4. Nachtrag 1985.

Homöopathisches Arzneibuch (Nachtrag zum HAB 1) 1991 1. Ausgabe. 1. Nachtrag zur Gesamtausgabe, zugleich 5. Nachtrag zur Ausgabe 1978. Amtliche Ausgabe, Deutscher Apothekerverlag Stuttgart, Govi-Verlag, Frankfurt

Kayne SB 1997 Homeopathic Pharmacy: an introduction and handbook. Churchill Livingstone, London

Keller K, Greiner S, Stockebrand P 1992 Homöopathische Arzneimittel. Materialien Zur Bewertung Aufbereitungsmonographien der Kommission D des deutschen Bundesgesundheitsamtes (BGA). Einschl. 4. Lieferung. Govi-Verlag, Frankfurt (Monograph collection, published by the German 'Bundesgesundheitsamt', BGA).

Melchart D, Wagner H 1993 Naturheilverfahren. Grundlagen einer autoregulativen Medizin. (Natural therapies. Basics of an autoregulative medicine. Schattauer, Stuttgart, pp 2–25.

Oxford Dictionary of English Etymology 1986 Oxford University Press, Oxford

Porter, R 1999 Greatest Benefit To Mankind: a medical history of humanity from antiquity to the present. Fontana, London

Resch G, Gutmann V 1987 Scientific Foundations Of Homoeopathy. Barthel & Barthel, Berg am Starnberger See

Stedmans Electronic Medical Dictionary 1998 (Version 4.0a). Williams and Wilkins, Baltimore

Taber's Cyclopaedic Medical Dictionary 1997 18th edn. Davis, Philadelphia

Yasgur's Homeopathic Dictionary and Holistic Health Reference 1998 Van Hoy, Philadelphia

Category Index

Categories

Biochemistry
Biography
Biophysics
Case taking and analysis
Constitution
Disease processes
Drug action
Healing processes
History
Materia medica
Medical methods

Morphology
Pathology
Pharmacology
Pharmacy
Philosophy
Physiology
Practitioner
Research
Symptomatology
Terrain
Therapeutics

b

C

d

r

S

t

Printed and bound by CPI Group (UK) Ltd, Croydon, CR0 4YY

14/10/2024

01773958-0001